MW00849023

Roopa Babannavar
Arvind Shenoy
Shitalkumar Sagari

Porcelain Laminate Veneers

Roopa Babannavar
Arvind Shenoy
Shitalkumar Sagari

Porcelain Laminate Veneers

Predictable and durable esthetic corrections for anterior teeth

LAP LAMBERT Academic Publishing

Imprint

Any brand names and product names mentioned in this book are subject to trademark, brand or patent protection and are trademarks or registered trademarks of their respective holders. The use of brand names, product names, common names, trade names, product descriptions etc. even without a particular marking in this work is in no way to be construed to mean that such names may be regarded as unrestricted in respect of trademark and brand protection legislation and could thus be used by anyone.

Cover image: www.ingimage.com

Publisher:
LAP LAMBERT Academic Publishing
is a trademark of
International Book Market Service Ltd., member of OmniScriptum Publishing Group
17 Meldrum Street, Beau Bassin 71504, Mauritius

Printed at: see last page
ISBN: 978-3-659-38967-2

Zugl. / Approved by: Davangere, Rajiv Gandhi University of Health Sciences, 2011

PORCELAIN LAMINATE VENEERS

Author: **Dr. Roopa Babannavar, MDS**
Co-authors: Dr. Arvind Shenoy, MDS
               Dr. Shitalkumar Sagari, MDS

1

Table of Contents

INTRODUCTION

People have long been fascinated by beauty. Throughout the world, beauty, glamour and positive self-image have always been considered desirable. A desire to look attractive is no longer taken as a sign of vanity. In an economically, socially and sexually competitive world; a pleasing appearance is a necessity. The face is the most recognizable feature of the body. Facial expressions mirror our emotional states and serve as crucial non-verbal communication tools.

"SMILE" is the most beautiful of all expressions. A smile has been said to be one of the most important interactive communication skills of a person. The ultimate objective of aesthetics in dentistry is to create a beautiful smile, with teeth of pleasing inherent proportions to one another, and a pleasing tooth arrangement in harmony with the gingiva, lips and face of the patient. [1]

The patients' demand for treatment of unaesthetic anterior teeth is steadily growing. Accordingly, several treatment options have been proposed to restore the aesthetic appearance of the dentition. This phenomenon has been both a bane and a boon to the dental profession. Rush-to-market products, media-driven treatment plans, as well as dentists eager to please, have formed a disquieting triad with little regard for the risk/benefit calculus of dental rehabilitation. On the other hand, new materials wedded to precise techniques have emerged to blur the interface between biologic and artificial structures. [2]

For many years, the most predictable and durable aesthetic correction of anterior teeth has been achieved by the preparation of full crowns. However, this approach is undoubtedly most invasive with substantial removal of large amounts of sound tooth substance and possible adverse effects on adjacent pulp and periodontal tissues. The great progress in bonding capability to both enamel and dentine made with the introduction of multi-step total-etch adhesive systems, along with the development of high performance and more universally applicable small particle hybrid resin composites has led to more conservative restorative adhesive techniques to deal with unaesthetic tooth appearance. Resin composite veneers can be used to mask tooth discolorations and/or to correct unaesthetic tooth forms and/or positions. [3]

However, such restorations still suffer from a limited longevity, because resin composites remain susceptible to discoloration, wear and marginal fractures, reducing thereby the aesthetic result in the long term. In search for more durable aesthetics, porcelain veneers have been introduced during the last decade. They are one of the most conservative and aesthetic techniques that we can apply when restoring the human dentition. In 1938, Dr Charles Pincus described a technique in which porcelain veneers were retained by a denture adhesive during cinematic filming. From the time of their introduction, till date the clinical and laboratory techniques have continued to be refined. [4]

Since their development 25 years ago, etched porcelain veneer restoration has proved to be a durable and aesthetic modality of treatment. These past 25 years of success can be attributed to great attention to detail in the following areas: (1) planning the case, (2) conservative (enamel saving) preparation of teeth, (3) proper selection of ceramics to use, (4) proper selection of the materials and methods of cementation of these restorations, (5) proper finishing and polishing of the restorations, and (6) proper planning for the continuing maintenance of these restorations. [5]

The strength of traditional porcelain is generally adequate for anterior porcelain veneers is supported by a number of clinical studies. Some authors have reported low rates of failure because of the loss of retention and fracture (0–5%) with short and medium term studies of up to

5

5 years. Indeed, long-term (15- and 20-year) retrospective studies indicated that the success rates of veneers are as high as 94% to 95% percent. These excellent results may, amongst other things, reflect careful case selection, but it is worth noting that other authors have reported much higher rates of failure of between 7–14% over 2–5 years. [6]

This dissertation summarizes the case selection, materials being used, various preparations and procedures involved, their merits and demerits, failures and the advancements in preparation approach.

HISTORICAL PERSPECTIVES

Glazed porcelain has a long history of use in dentistry as one of the most esthetic and biocompatible materials available, surpassed only by enamel itself.

The advent of porcelain labial veneers as a permanent esthetic restoration marked the progression of more than 30 years of dental research in acid etch, bonding and esthetic restorative techniques.[7]

In 1938, Dr. Charles Pincus, was the first person to use a denture adhesive to bond thin temporary veneers to teeth. It was done to enhance actor's appearance for close – ups in the movie industry.[8]

Rochette, in1975 described the innovative restoration of a fractured incisor with an "etched silanated porcelain block". He baked a ceramic block in the lab on a 24- karat gold matrix cast. A resin was bonded to the silane treated porcelain block & etched enamel. [7]

Porcelain veneers bonded to etched enamel evolved from this technique and became popular in Europe through the work of Touti et al. [8]

In 1982, Simonsen & Calamia demonstrated good bond strengths for resin composite to hydrofluoric acid etched porcelain & that the use of a silane coupling agent could further increase the bond strength of a resin composite to etched porcelain.

Horn introduced the platinum foil technique in early 1900's.

Other methods such as pressed (ex: IPS Empress) or a castable ceramic (Dicor) and CAD/CAM (ex: Cerec) or copy milling techniques (ex: Celay) have also been developed for porcelain veneer fabrication. [9]

CASE SELECTION

INDICATIONS- According to Pascal Magne [8]

He divided the indications into 3 principal groups

Type I- tooth discoloration resistant to bleaching procedure

    IA- tetracycline discoloration of degree III & IV

    IB- no response to external/ internal bleaching

Type II- the need for major morphologic modification in anterior teeth

    IIA- conoid teeth

    IIB- diastemata & interdental triangles to be closed

    IIC- augmentation of incisal length & prominence

Type III- extensive restoration of compromised anterior teeth

    IIIA- extensive coronal fracture

    IIIB- extensive loss of enamel by resorption & wear

    IIIC- generalized congenital & acquired malformation

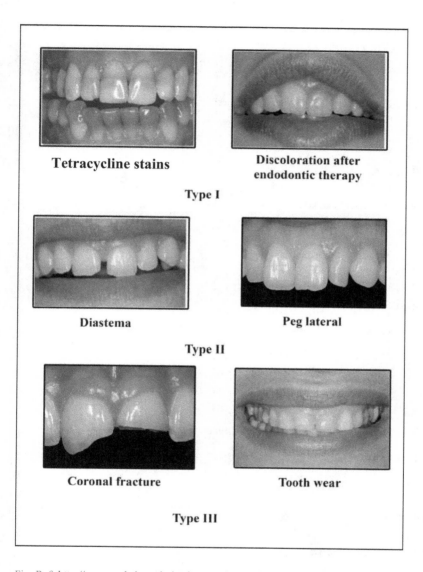

Tetracycline stains

Discoloration after
endodontic therapy

Type I

Diastema

Peg lateral

Type II

Coronal fracture

Tooth wear

Type III

By Ching Chiat Lim [10]

1. Management of non carious surface defects

   -Localized enamel malformations- Eroded teeth

   - Enamel hypocalcifications

   -Hypoplasia

2. Masking of discolorations

   - Fluorosis
   - Tetracycline staining
   - Necrosis

3. Repair of structural defects

   - Fractured incisal edges
   - Mild malalignment of teeth
   - Closure of diastemas
   - Peg shaped lateral incisors

4. Repair of fractured porcelain facings on fixed prosthesis

5. Replacement of old resin composite veneers

6. Orthodontic retainers

Contraindications

By Roger Smales, Frederick Chu [9]

1. Insufficient amount of enamel for bonding

   - Extensive caries

- Tooth fractures

- Heavily restored teeth

- Severe enamel hypoplasia

- Short clinical crowns

2. Excessive forces acting on teeth

   - Bruxism

   - Object biting habits

3. Malocclusion, extensive periodontal bone loss

DIAGNOSTIC APPROACH &

TREATMENT PLANNING

Esthetic dentistry is functional, biocompatible, and ultimately attractive, but at the same time complex and demanding.

This reflects the importance of diagnosis and treatment planning in any esthetic procedures including porcelain veneers. The treatment outcome of porcelain veneers strongly depends on the therapeutic approach chosen.

Criteria for case selection-

According to Ching Chiat Lim [10]

1. Static & dynamic occlusal relationship-

Determining the occlusal relation dictates through various procedural steps of veneer preparation. The incisal porcelain finishing line is determined by the contact relationship between the incisors and canines in centric & eccentric position.

The margin should be placed so that they do not contact the opposing dentition during the rest position. Ideally, occlusal contacts during the centric position & lateral excursion should be on porcelain or tooth structure completely.

Occlusal interferences and parafunctional habits are contraindications for porcelain veneers as they'll result in crack formation and eventual fracture of restoration.

2. Periodontal and oral health status

Healthy periodontium facilitates impression taking, cementation, and maintenance. Hence patient's overall periodontal and oral health status should be evaluated.

Mouth breathers have poor oral gingival health, hence poor candidates for porcelain veneers.

3. Condition of tooth

- Degree of discoloration

If tooth is grossly discolored, bleaching of the tooth first before veneer is placed should be considered.

In teeth with tetracycline staining, discoloration becomes more evident as enamel is reduced. These should be masked using opaque glass ionomer cement or opaque porcelain.

- Extent of caries

After caries removal if little or no enamel is left, porcelain veneer placement is contraindicated. This is because; the veneer- tooth complex is weakened when the surface area of enamel available for bonding is decreased by 50%.

- Extent of restoration

If present, the restoration should be small enough that the area for bonding with enamel is not compromised.

The old restorations should be replaced if there is a questionable status for underlying caries.

- Quality of tooth

Structural defects, such as amelogenesis imperfecta and dentinogenesis imperfecta which leave insufficient enamel and tooth structure for bonding are definite contraindication for veneers.

4. Oral habits-

Presence of oral habits such as nail or pencil biting is a contraindication for veneer as the shear stress may be too great for the ceramics to withstand.

According to Pascal Magne [8]

The initial phase of diagnosis and treatment planning should be of following sequence

1. Know the patient

   It aims to understand the patient's primary request.

2. Initial documentation

   It includes a radiographic survey and a systematic clinical examination (evaluation of periodontal and endodontic conditions, existing restorations, etc). Photographs and study casts, possibly mounted in an articulator, complete the initial documentation.

3. Inform the patient

   The clinician can explain the existing problems to the patient, using the radiographs, photographs, and study models as aids. The major elements of the treatment options are explained.

4. Sequential treatment plan

   Duration and costs are determined.

5. Initial patient management

   Once the patient gives informed consent, the practical modalities of the treatment can be planned. The initial phase of treatment typically comprises preventive, periodontal, and operative aspects, which are usually neglected.

The following interventions are most frequently undertaken when esthetics plays a key role: mucogingival surgery, bleaching, orthodontics, and direct composite restorations.

Mucogingival surgery

Adequate health and morphology of the periodontium are responsible for 50% of the final esthetic outcome. In some situations, graft-type interventions or minor remodeling of gingival contours can ensure the final outcome of the restorations.

Bleaching

The optical conditions of underlying dental tissues can have a negative influence on the final esthetics; bleaching procedures allow reestablishment of a tooth color that will facilitate integration of the bonded porcelain restorations. The restorative phase must be delayed for 2 to 4 weeks after the end of bleaching because of the inhibiting effect of oxygen residues on the bond strength of composites.

Orthodontics and orthognathic surgery- Realignment of teeth to be veneered is generally undertaken before the restorative phase. In some rare cases, orthognathic surgery might be indicated in conjunction with orthodontics, which requires special treatment planning.

Direct composites

Minor modifications of neighboring teeth are often necessary before placing veneers. A typical situation is the optimization of lateral incisor shape and volume before veneering central incisors.

According to **Dino Javaheri,** [11] depending on the existing conditions and the desired result, clinicians have to plan preparation techniques for porcelain veneers:

1. No preparation
2. Enamel-only preparation
3. Varied levels of dentin preparation
4. Interproximal extensions

MATERIALS USED

Choice Of Ceramic Material For Manufacturing Porcelain Laminate Veneers According To Clinical Indication

Patients can be divided according to whether the veneers will be subjected to functional loading or not:

(a) Type I patients

(b) Type II patients

Type I patients-

In these cases the facets are not exposed to functional loading, and are referred to as simple esthetic facets.

These patients are candidates for conventional ceramics.

They are classified into two subgroups according to the background color characteristics of the treated teeth.

(a) Type I-A patients: these are subjects programmed to receive simple esthetic facets were the substrate teeth present no color alterations. The only objective in this case is to apply PLVs for shape modifying purposes.

(b) Type I-B patients: these patients are likewise programmed to receive simple esthetic facets, though in this case the substrate teeth present color alterations. Therefore, and independently of the need for shape modifications, the selected ceramic material must be able to hide the underlying substrate color.

Type II patients-

In these cases the facets are exposed to functional loading, and are referred to as functional esthetic facets.

These patients require high resistance ceramics.

Once the patients programmed for porcelain facet treatment have been classified, the dental porcelain material best suited to the physical and optic requirements of each case, based on the above described material classification is chosen.

Type I-A patients

Patients with facets that will not be subjected to functional loading and present a clear substrate
The material used only aims to solve problems relating to tooth shape
These are consequently favorable cases, since only a small ceramic material thickness is required. In these situations conventional feldspate ceramics are recommended for use, in view of their excellent optic characteristics that afford optimum esthetic results.
The absence of occlusal stress in these cases, and the use of the currently available adhesion contribute to ensure prolonged restoration survival.
Problem is posed in medium or large (over 2 mm) interincisal diastema cases. In this setting it must be taken into account that as the porcelain extends beyond the adhesion zone, it loses the "protective" increase in elastic modulus afforded by the adhesion and composite resin. In these patients the use of high resistance feldspate ceramics is recommended – since their good esthetic qualities combine with adequate resistance to fracture.

Type I-B patients

These patients' present facets that will not bear functional loading but which show moderate to severe alterations in dental color that must be effectively masked by the restoration. In these situations both the porcelain and cement must present various degrees of opacity in order to hide the color alterations and this in turn implies problems to secure the desired optic effects in terms of translucency and reflectance, and consequently also esthetic outcome.

Tooth preparation will be more aggressive (0.8-1 mm), and the finishing line should be slightly subgingival and involving a curved chamfer in order to increase the ceramic thickness and prevent an overlay notorious tooth-restoration transition zone.

Type II patients

In these cases the existence of functional loading in both the mandibular static position and during excursive movements requires the use of a material with great resistance to fracture. Accordingly, feldspate or alumina ceramics of high resistance, and oxide ceramics are indicated. Consequently, the use of high resistance ceramics with the lost-wax casting technique is recommended. (IPS Empress II, Style Press, IPS Empress I, Optec HSP, Mirage, Finesse, Cergogold y Empress esthetic), because of its esthetic properties and predictability, in long term studies, in the oral rehabilitation of the anterior guide.[12]

Feldspates-

- The predominant element in this case is silica oxide or quartz in a proportion of 46-66% versus 11-17% of alumina.
- The feldspate porcelains in turn are sub classified as follows: Conventional feldspate porcelains & High resistance feldspate porcelains.

Conventional feldspate porcelains

- These offer very good esthetic effects but the main problem is that they are fragile (low fracture resistance: 56.5 MPa).

- Ex- Vintage, Luxor, Duceram, Flexoceram, Vivodent PE, IPS Classic, Empress esthetic

High resistance feldspate porcelains

(a) Feldspate porcelain reinforced with leucite crystals.

- The chemical composition in this case comprises quartz (68%) and aluminum oxide (18%). As a result of the pressing process used to manufacture these materials, porosity is reduced and adequate and reproducible fit precision is achieved. The perfect distribution of the leucite crystals within the glass matrix, observable during the cooling phase and after pressing, contributes to increase resistance without significantly diminishing translucency.

- The resistance to flexion is 160-300 MPa.

- Examples of this type of porcelain include IPS-Empress I, Optec HSP, Mirage, Finesse, Cergogold.

(b) Feldspate porcelain reinforced with lithium oxide.

- The chemical composition in this case comprises quartz (57-80%), lithium oxide (11-19%) and aluminum oxide (0-5%).

- The incorporation of these crystalline particles increases the flexion resistance to 320-450 MPa.[13]

PRESSABLE CERAMICS

IPS Empress. This is a type of feldspathic porcelain supplied in ingot form. The ingots are heated and molded under pressure to produce the restorations. A full-contour crown is waxed, invested and placed in a specialized mold that has an alumina plunger. The ceramic ingot is placed under the plunger, the entire assembly is heated to 1150^0 C and the plunger presses the molten ceramic into the mold. The final shade of the crown is adjusted by staining or veneering.

Optec OPC is also a type of feldspathic porcelain with increased leucite content, processed by molding under pressure and heat. The OPC system can be used for full-contour restorations (inlays, veneers, full crowns). Both Optec OPC and IPS Empress produce strong, translucent, dense and etchable ceramic restorations. The materials are especially useful in fabricating ceramic veneers. Both systems require special equipment (pressing oven and die material) to fabricate the restorations.[14]

ADVANTAGES OF

PRESSED CERAMIC:

- Wear compatibility
- Increased translucency
- Ability to wax-up final contours prior to pressing
- Stronger than feldspathic (IPS Empress 120 MPa compared to 60 MPa to110 MPa feldspathic)
- More consistent results for the average ceramist

ADVANTAGES OF FELDSPATHIC CERAMIC:

- Ability to mask out darker preps

- Less tooth structure removal (.3 mm to .5 mm vs. .6 mm to .8 mm)

- More 3D appearance in thinner areas

- Ability to use same ceramic as in adjacent PFMs

- Ability to place different opacity levels within the restoration

RECOMMENDATIONS FOR PRESSED CERAMIC SELECTION:

- When significant malposition exists in arch

- When significant increase in tooth length is desired

- When strength is of utmost importance

RECOMMENDATIONS FOR FELDSPATHIC CERAMIC SELECTION:

- When minimal preparation is desired due to patient concerns or minimal changes in size, shape, and shade

- Diastema closures when shade is not altered significantly

- Teeth with minimal malpositions within the arch

- When adjacent teeth will have PFM restorations placed [15]

Common Restorative Materials for Dental CAD/CAM System [16]

Restorative Material	CAD/CAM System	Indications	Adhesive Cementation	Conventional Cementation	Flexural Strength
Dicor MCG (fluormica)	Cerec	Inlays, onlays, veneers	Yes, dual-cured	No	< 100 MPa
Vita Mark II (feldspathic)	Cerec	Inlays, onlays, veneers, anterior crowns	Yes, dual-cured	No	150 MPa
ProCAD (leucite-reinforced)	Cerec	Inlays, onlays, veneers, anterior crowns	Yes, dual-cured	No	150 MPa

PRE-OPERATIVE EVALUATION

Various predetermining factors play important roles in the evaluation and decision-making process of the treatment planning of each case. In cases where PLVs are planned, many factors should be thoroughly determined before the actual treatment begins. These details must be carefully analyzed to minimize difficult situations that may arise during the actual treatment process and to avoid possible postoperative complications.

To select the most appropriate option for each patient, the dentist must carefully evaluate each case, review all available options, and clearly define how that goal will be reached, along with what necessary steps must be followed in order to achieve the desired result. The dentist must first examine and evaluate each tooth and its surrounding tissues to ensure that they are functionally sufficient. Once this is established, careful attention to a functional diagnosis should be made, leading to the definition of reconstructive goals for both the dentist and his/her technical staff. Clear goals are essential to avoid any misunderstanding that could compromise the esthetic results, and when fully understood by all parties involved, the chances for success are greatly increased.[17]

The Face

The face is the first view requiring assessment by a dental practitioner. This view not only reveals the physical landmarks of a person's identity, but also gives clues to their psychological make-up or persona. Facial expressions mirror our emotional states and serve as crucial non-verbal communication tools. Depending on the surrounding soft tissue envelope of the lips and cheeks, showing anterior teeth can signify pleasure (by a smile), or disdain (by a sneer). These examples illustrate the importance of teeth to the facial composition, serving the functions of mastication, communication and social interaction. Consequently, analysis of facial features influences dental restorations, particularly in the anterior region, by integrating with existing skeletal and soft tissue features to either enhance desirable qualities or distract attention from undesirable abnormalities.

The facial composition is one of the most important issues for the patient. This perspective influences most patients' notions of a perfect smile.

Various ways of facial assessment

- Physiognomonic
- Morpho psychological
- Geometric

Physiognomy

It's the art of judging an individual's character or personality by the appearance of their face.

Morphopsychology-

It involves in establishing a link between the morphology of the human body with the psychological makeup. Facial analysis is assessed by the following factors-

- Facial typology
- Facial zones & segmental expansion
- Sensitive receptors
- Tegumental texture & relief
- Sexual type

GEOMETRIC-

It is method of facial assessment based on mathematical principles of evaluating beauty.

A geometric evaluation of the face is visualizing imaginary lines in the frontal and sagittal views. Starting from the upper to the lower parts of the face, the horizontal lines are:

- Hair
- Opharic
- Interpupillary
- Interalar
- Commissural

These parallel lines create horizontal symmetry and act as cohesive forces unifying the facial composition. The facial midline is perpendicular to the horizontal lines and opposes their cohesiveness. These are called as segregative force and are essential in a composition to give interest and harmony. The cohesive forces are paramount in achieving pleasing esthetics.

The interpupillary line is used as a reference for the occlusal and the incisal plane orientations. [1]

DENTOFACIAL PERSPECTIVE-

This perspective concentrates on the orofacial landmarks consisting of highly vascularised lips with the teeth acting as a gateway to the oral cavity.

The Lips-

In static position of lips four factors influence tooth exposure: lip length, age, race and sex, also known as the acronym L A R S.

LIP LENGTH- It influences the amount of tooth visibility. Individuals with long maxillary lips show more mandibular than maxillary teeth.

AGE- The amount of maxillary tooth displayed is inversely proportional to increasing age, whereas the amount of mandibular teeth directly proportional to increasing age.

RACE- A decreasing amount of maxillary, and an increasing amount of mandibular tooth visibility, is seen from Caucasians to Asians to Blacks.

SEX- Males generally have longer maxillary lips than females, leading to an average maxillary tooth display of 1.91 mm for men and 3.40 mm for women (twice the display).

The dynamic position of lips is characterized by a smile. The extent of tooth exposure during a smile depends on skeletal make-up, degree of contraction of the facial muscles, shape and size of the dental elements and shape and size of the lips.

Lips vary from extremely thin to full and thick. According to Rufenacht's morph psychological concepts, individuals with thin and taut lips should be provided with teeth which confer delicacy and fragility. Conversely, patients endowed with thick or voluptuous lips require teeth which display dominance and boldness.

The cohesive forces are created by parallelism of the incisal and commissural lines, with the segregative force of the dental midline intersecting at 90 degrees.

The Smile Line

The smile line is an imaginary line running from the incisal edges of the maxillary incisors and coinciding with the curvature of the lower lip. It is often lost due to wear by abrasion, erosion or attrition, periodontitis, altered patterns of eruption or poor quality dentistry. [18]

DENTAL PERSPECTIVE-

The dental perspective concerns the teeth, their shape, size, intra- and inter-arch relationships.[19]

Tooth position

In-depth knowledge of the hard tissues of the mouth and the teeth is essential to the development of restorative procedures. Biomimetics, one of the new terms introduced to the dental glossary by Magne, et al., refers to the reproduction of the original performance of the intact tooth that is about to be restored. This is vitally important when restoring fractured, worn-out or aged teeth. In most cases, even if the teeth are intact, their improper alignment, rotation, lingual labial position will play an important role in treatment planning (see aesthetic pre-recontouring), as the amount of sound tooth reduction is often related to the position of the teeth. For example, the extreme labial position of the tooth must be more aggressively prepared than the facial in order to keep the finished PLV level with the rest of the arch. Pulp status (for example, pulp size in a young patient) should be evaluated and, in lingually aligned teeth, care must be taken not to reduce unnecessarily the facial structure of the tooth. [17]

The factors to be evaluated in individual tooth are-
- Hue
- Value, Chroma, & Translucency
- Surface texture & luster

Tooth shape-
- Size of tooth (height : width ratio)
- Incisal edge contour
- Shape of the tooth
- Analysis of static
- Spatial arrangement of teeth [20]

Gingiva

The soft tissues and bone height in relation to adjacent teeth should always be taken into account to avoid gingival asymmetry and to maintain the height of the interdental papillae. If this is not carefully evaluated, the formation of black holes at the gingival embrasures will be unavoidable, and in some cases may even be the cause of a variety of problems. This is especially true if it has not been discussed with the patient before the treatment begins. Poor dental hygiene, gingival inflammation and one or more gingival recession sites should all be treated. It is even more crucial that patients are observed for a period of time in order to determine the extent of the cooperation exhibited.

Gingival Margins

The cervical placement of the PLV margins is also an important issue to be taken into consideration. Although the laminate veneer's ideal margins are preferably located on the enamel and away from the gingiva, the condition of the teeth must always be appraised before deciding on any form of treatment. The extent of previous restorations and carious lesions, defective enamel or gingival recession and root exposure, especially in the case of a high lip-line, may necessitate the overextension of the preparation margins, and special care should be exercised in doing so. The incisal edge position sets the starting point of the esthetic treatment planning, as discussed before. Therefore, to avoid unesthetic or unpredictable results, the crown length, incisal wear, and the extent of the lengthening of the incisal aspect should be carefully evaluated and only then should the extent of gingival alterations be decided.

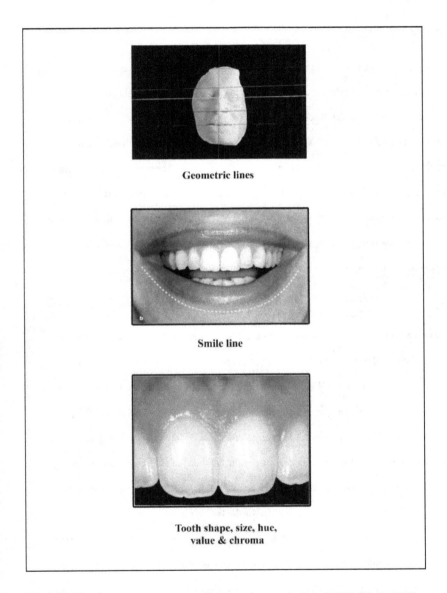

Geometric lines

Smile line

**Tooth shape, size, hue,
value & chroma**

Fig- I. Ahmad. Anterior dental esthetics: Facial perspective Br Dent J 2005;199 (1): 15-21

35

Occlusion

Occlusal relations, heavy function or parafunction play vital roles in PLV applications. In some cases, where the patient exhibits severe parafunctional habits or unfavorable occlusal relations, full ceramic or porcelain-fused-to-metal crowns may be considered the preferred choice for restoring these teeth. It is a well-known fact that cervical abfractions, specifically at the premolars, are due to tooth flexing under heavy occlusal forces. These are some of the clues to heavy occlusion that have to be very carefully evaluated before any definitive restorative treatment is undertaken. The relative fragility of PLV restorations requires an accurate analysis of the patient's occlusion, to ensure that the restorations do not extend into areas of occlusal stress. The results of this analysis may limit the opportunities for remodeling.

Age

Aged or worn-out teeth exhibit different thicknesses of enamel and surface texture that are directly related to the extent and distribution of the occlusal interferences or external stimuli. While treating such cases with PLVs the most important issue is not the strength of the ceramic material, which has been proven to be three times stronger than the enamel in tensile strength, but the preservation of sufficient enamel and controlling the occlusal forces. In the aged tooth, the enamel may be so thin that any extra preparation for PLV may lead to a loss of this existing precious enamel, while the loss of the surface area of etchable enamel may directly affect bonding. An even more critical issue, perhaps, is the loss of the thickness of this enamel that is so vitally related to the flexibility of the tooth. The thinner the enamel gets, the more flexible the teeth become. In order to avoid this and to maintain the natural strength of the tooth, preserving the already existing enamel is of prime importance, especially while working with the aged tooth.

The strength of the bonded veneer, together with the preserved existing enamel, will minimize the tooth flex and thus create a strong bond between the PLV and the enamel.[17]

PROCEDURE

ARMAMENTARIUM

It is the shape of the instrument that determines the profile of the preparation. TPS (Touati) Brasseler kits were introduced in 1985. This instrument kit consists of eight burs, enabling veneer preparations to be accomplished in total safety. The laminate veneer preparation kit comprises:

- Two instruments (gauges TFC1 and TFC2) to monitor labial reduction;
- Two instruments (TFC3 and TFC4) for reduction of enamel and margins;
- Two instruments (TFC5 and TFC6) for occlusal reduction;
- Two instruments (TFC7 and TFC8) for finishing.

The advantage of this kit lies in simplifying preparation by plain codifying and offering a limited number of instruments.

The two depth-cutter instruments (TFC1, TFC2) serve to guide, visualize and, in particular, quantify enamel reduction. In addition, margins can be plotted, owing to the rounded tip. The manufactures consider it dangerous to gauge reduction in enamel depth of between 0.3 and 0.5 mm without some type of depth guide. [20]

Another instrument kit that is available is LVS i.e. Laminate Veneer System (Brasseler, Savannah, Ga.) it contains two depth-cutting diamond that come in two sizes (LVS no. 1 and LVS no. 2). [7]

Simple round diamond burs represent ideal depth cutters. The depth of cut (DC) is easily calculated with formula by measuring the diameter of the bur (d1) and the diameter of the shank (d2). A DC of 0.5 mm is recommended for cervical preparations and 0.7 mm for the incisal two-thirds. [21]

The primary preparation design for porcelain veneers, also called bonded laminates or bonded porcelain restorations (BPRs), should simultaneously allow an ideal marginal adaptation of the final restoration and reflect an optimal adaptation of the hard tissue morphology. A minimum amount of preparation geometry is required to facilitate insertion and positioning of the ceramic restoration during the final bonding procedure. The geometric and mechanical parameters of the tooth preparation, however, are of only secondary importance. This allows for maximal preservation of remaining sound mineralized tissue during the tooth preparation procedure and, consequently, a conservative approach (i.e., approximately one-quarter the amount of tooth reduction of conventional complete-coverage crowns; One essential goal—the long-term presentation of the tooth-restoration complex—requires the achievement of a sufficient ceramic thickness to provide the restoration with some intrinsic mechanical resistance.

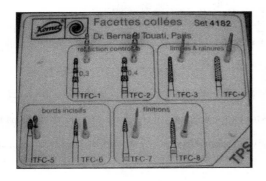

Laminate veneer preparation kit

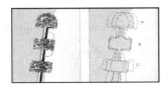

Depth cutter

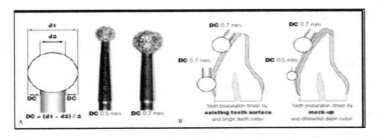

Fig- Ref- Touti B, Miara P & Nathanson D. Esthetic dentistry & ceramic restorations. Martin Dunitz.

GUREL G. The science & art of porcelain laminate veneers. Quint pub.

PASCAL MAGNE, URS C. BELSER. Novel Porcelain Laminate Preparation Approach Driven by a Diagnostic Mock-Up. J Esthet Restor Dent 16:7–18, 2004

MOCK UP

To get a better idea instantly of what the eventual outcome will be, utilization of the composite mock-up is wonderful as an aid. The neighboring tissues or teeth provide three-dimensional information that is necessary to give the restoration the correct volume and shape. A diagnostic "composite mock-up" which is the direct application of composite without surface preparation that perches itself on the teeth, is indicated when such elements are missing, or when an alteration of tooth forms is necessary.

Determining the Incisal Edge Position

It gives the patient an inexpensive preview of what the veneer will look like. Without these visual aids, it is difficult for even the most experienced dentist to predict the final outcome. It enables the dentist to establish the incisal length of the centrals as well as the buccal-lingual position of the incisal edge and the incisal edge plane. It is also helpful in establishing the lateral, central incisor relationship and their axial inclinations.

Determining the Gingival Line

A trial that can be referred to as a "reverse mockup" is also possible to make. If the dentist decides that the incisal edge positions of the teeth are in their correct place, but that the teeth still appear short, this may be an indication for alteration of the gingival levels. In such a case, instead of adding the composite material over the incisal edge, the material is added over the gingiva after it has been dried. This will appear a little over contoured since the composite is being added over the original volume of the gingiva. However, it offers the patient a great chance to visualize and to formulate an idea about the appearance of the new smile and of the longer teeth that have been lengthened towards the apical direction. Once the patient is satisfied with the new appearance, an alginate impression can be made from this mock-up and sent to the lab. After this, a transparent template can be built which can be used as a surgical stand, to dictate where the new gingiva should be located. This will serve as an indispensable communicative tool to the periodontologist who will be responsible for altering the gingival levels.

Interactive Patient Communication

These composite mock-ups can also be used to open a discussion with the patient as to how their smile can be modified. Here the finer details of the restoration, such as the nuances of color and all pertinent parameters - position, contour and proper communication - can be tested and given approval by the patient.

The dentist should use the mock-up, if not for any other reason, just for the wonderful educational and enlightening experience it offers the patient. [17]

Technique

The easiest way of doing the mockup is with the freehand carving method. The composite is rolled between the fingers and applied over the dried tooth structure. It is shaped with the help of the fingers and special hand carving instruments and then light cured. The teeth can be lengthened or protruded, or the color can be altered for the patient to visualize. After placing the composite mock-up on the tooth, if any part is over exaggerated, it can be corrected with the help of a fissure diamond bur.

Advantages of tooth preparation

Correct tooth preparation initiates control of the following:

1.		Contour
	a.	Emergence angle
	b.	Margin
	c.	Facial profile
2.		Color without overbulking
3.		Margin placement for concealment
4.		Veneer seating for placement and bonding
5.		Definitiveness of margin for the technician
6.		Porcelain bulk for occlusal loading
7.		Glaze preservation in finishing procedures
8.		Tooth recontouring for misalignment correction
9.		Enamel etch by removing fluoride- rich layer [17]

Various basic principles of tooth preparation for veneers

1) Tooth preparation should remain wherever possible in enamel.

2) Sufficient thickness of porcelain should be present to allow masking of any underlying tooth discoloration without the need to overbuild tooth contour.

3) The preparation should result in a smooth transition between tooth and restoration and in the gingival region should maintain the correct emergence profile.

4) Restoration margins should not be placed in positions where there is a high degree of occlusal loading.

5) Sharp line angles should be avoided to prevent the propagation of undesirable stress fractures in the bonded ceramic material. [22]

Tooth-preparation techniques can be divided in two groups according to their underlying principles:

- Those driven by the existing tooth surface,
- Those driven by the final volume of the preparation.

Preparation Driven by Existing Tooth Surface

In techniques driven by the existing tooth surface, the ultimate goal is to remove a uniform layer of the tooth structure. This can be achieved by freehand preparation using traditional diamond burs (round ended and slightly tapered) and silicone guides of the existing tooth. The same objective can be attained by using depth cutters (e.g., burs with calibrated diamond rings), which is a more accurate and time-efficient strategy. In this approach there are reduced diagnostic steps and limited communication with the dental laboratory technician because the intrinsic principle is the reproduction of the initial situation (in terms of form and function). This approach can be recommended only after a careful preoperative evaluation of the case, confirming the integrity of the original enamel thickness and knowledge that the final goal of the restoration will be limited to the reproduction of the existing tooth volume, shape, and function. Such cases are rare and typically involve patients with intact discolored teeth that are not responding to bleaching (i.e. indicated for BPRs type I, according to Magne and Belser).

Preparation Driven by Final Volume of Restoration

These cases require a specific diagnostic approach and require a high level of communication with the dental laboratory technician. In these cases the BPR aims to restore the original (not the existing) volume of the tooth, especially in the presence of thin initial enamel. Such cases typically involve patients with altered existing tooth shape (i.e., indicated for BPR types II and III, according to Magne and Belser). A diagnostic wax-up that represents the original volume of the tooth should be used as a reference for tooth reduction. This basic principle saves a significant amount of sound hard tissue, not just enamel but also the critical dentin-enamel junction. The simplest and most important tool for enamel reduction in this technique is represented by a well adapted horizontally sectioned silicone index from an additive wax-up. This method, however, can be time consuming.

New Simplified Technique

This new technique avoids the shortcomings of existing methods, simultaneously combining their related advantages: time efficiency, enamel preservation, subsequent improvement of adhesion and mechanics, and utmost respect of the pulp. Before proceeding with the tooth preparation sequence, the bonded acrylic mock-up is used by the patient for several days or weeks to ensure that the objective represented by the wax up is compatible with the individual's personality, face, smile, oral functions, and subjective expectations. Only after the patient's approval or objectively justified modification of the mockup configuration the tooth preparations are achieved.

Detailed Procedures

- Addition of wax onto the preliminary model

- Fabricating the corresponding acrylic template directly in the patient's mouth using self-curing resin molded on the existing tooth surfaces with a silicone matrix of the wax-up

- For optimal stability the silicone must overlap two teeth on each side of the modified segment. Palatal surfaces must remain accessible to allow the early elimination of palatal excess resin. The facial aspect of the matrix is then sectioned and ground to follow the contour of the scalloped gingival sulcus.

- Existing enamel is etched partially for 5 to 10 seconds rinsed, and dried to secure retention for the acrylic resin.

- Fill the silicone matrix partially with a dentin-type liquid acrylic resin; wait until the resin surface becomes dull in appearance.

- The index is then applied to the teeth and maintained in position while all accessible areas are cleared of excess resin. Increase the color saturation of interdental spaces using brownish light-curing stains to visually "break" the bonded connection between teeth.

- The final luster can be obtained by glazing with a very-low-viscosity resin.

- The mock-up should not be modified prior to completion of an assessment of 1 to 2 weeks, which is the usual elapsed time required for "deprogramming" of the patient from the previous situation.

- Tooth preparation procedures can be initiated upon agreement of the patient on the final objective, which can be easily assessed through the mock-up.

- A single horizontal groove of depth of 0.7mm is obtained and marked with a pencil at the junction of incisal third and middle third.

- A groove of depth 0.5mm is obtained which is slightly scalloped and later marked with pencil.

- The remaining part of the mock-up can be removed. This is followed by the use of traditional burs until the pencil marks are completely removed. A palatal index is used to assess the 1.5 mm incisal clearance

- The preparation is then finished. All transition line angles are finally rounded with flexible disks at a low speed

- Identification of possible dentin exposures and subsequent sealing of these areas with a dentin adhesive [21]

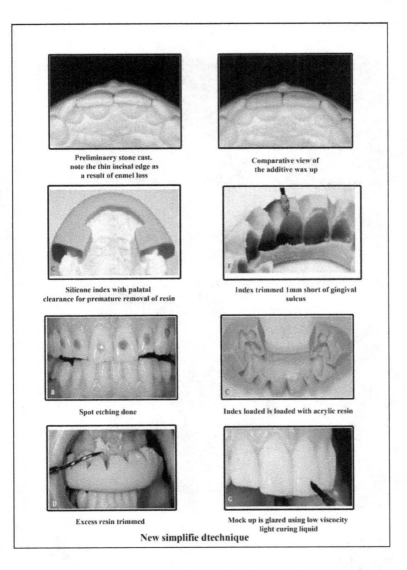

Preliminaery stone cast.
note the thin incisal edge as
a result of enmel loss

Comparative view of
the additive wax up

Silicone index with palatal
clearance for premature removal of resin

Index trimmed 1mm short of gingival
sulcus

Spot etching done

Index loaded is loaded with acrylic resin

Excess resin trimmed

Mock up is glazed using low viscocity
light curing liquid

New simplifie dtechnique

Fig- Ref- PASCAL MAGNE, URS C. BELSER. Novel Porcelain Laminate Preparation Approach Driven by a Diagnostic Mock-Up. J Esthet Restor Dent 16:7–18, 2004

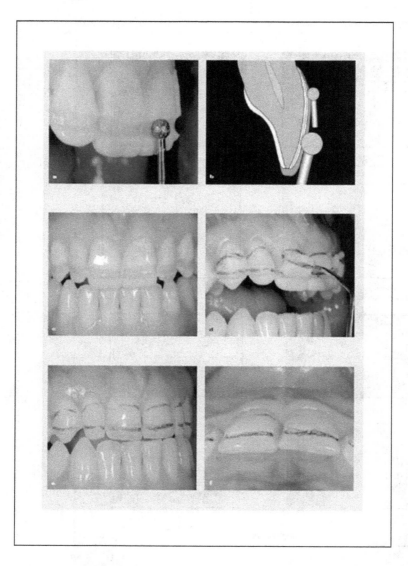

Fig- Ref- PASCAL MAGNE, URS C. BELSER. Novel Porcelain Laminate Preparation Approach Driven by a Diagnostic Mock-Up. J Esthet Restor Dent 16:7–18, 2004

TOOTH PREPARATION

Graded tooth preparation rests on the principle that the greater the color change, the greater the misalignment toward the facial, or the greater the occlusal function, the greater the amount of tooth reduction.

Two levels of graded tooth preparation are necessary to create space:

1. For a moderate color change (the universal preparation)
2. For profound color change.

For moderate color change, defined as two shades or less, a two plane facial reduction of 0.3mm in the cervical one third and 0.5mm in the incisal two thirds is indicated. This is called the universal preparation because more than 90% of the cases necessitate this preparation.

For profound color change, defined as 3 shades or more, including tetracycline and endodontically discolored teeth, a deeper biplane facial reduction is desirable. Mandibular incisors cannot be reduced more than 0.3mm cervically and 0.5mm on the remaining facial surface without substantial dentin exposure. [23]

Tooth preparation for maxillary anterior teeth

Before initiating tooth preparation, it is necessary to determine where to place the gingival margin. The advantages of a slightly supragingival margin (0.5 mm) are numerous, such as minimal tissue trauma in preparation, lessened likelihood of exposing dentin, reduced probability of tissue retraction for impression taking, greater control of surface contamination during bonding, easier access for marginal finishing procedures after placement, reduced probability of contour alterations in the bonded restoration (potentiating gingival inflammation), and improved patient accessibility for soft tissue maintenance. Therefore, with the exception of pronounced

51

tooth discoloration or a patient who is obsessive about disguising the margin, it is highly desirable to place the margin slightly supragingival in enamel. In cases in which a 0.5-mm supragingival margin has been prepared, as previously stated, placement of retraction cord is usually unnecessary.

Tooth preparation sequence: Maxillary teeth

To control the depth of the facial tooth preparation and remain primarily in enamel for bond strength and reliability of marginal seal, self-limiting, depth-cutting disks are used. These depth-cutting disks permit 0.3-mm, 0.5-mm, and 0.7-mm cuts to be placed anywhere on the facial surface

Placement of depth cuts

The 0.3-mm depth-cutting disk (or infrequently the 0.5-mm depth-cutting disk for profound color change) is used first to place a uniform horizontal depth cuts in the cervical one third of tooth.

Two more horizontal depth cuts are placed; one midfacially and another in the incisal one third of facial surface (0.5mm or 0.7mm depth cutting disk).

Gingivoproximal preparation

Using a long, tapered medium or fine grit snub-nosed diamond bur, a definitive chamfer (0.3 to 0.4 mm in depth) is prepared uniformly 0.5 mm supragingival from the gingival margin.

Margin placement begins at the height of the free gingival margin and continues to the distal papilla tip. Then the chamfer margin is prepared to the mesial papilla tip.

Preparation is taken far enough lingually, to hide the veneer margin when viewed from the side of the tooth. This produces an elbow-like cut, which translates into the "wings" of the forthcoming veneer, which will conceal the margin from an unaesthetic display

The tooth contact is left intact with a narrow island (0.2 mm) of proximal tooth structure labial to the contact zone, remaining unprepared.

The purpose of establishing the entire gingivoproximal definitive chamfer margin before beginning facial depth cut removal is to avoid over preparation, which often occurs when facial reduction is begun first.[23]

Depth of chamfer

This Gingivoproximal preparation can be shallow, medium or deep. If the chamfer is kept too deep then the replacing porcelain will be thicker than it should be and the thicker porcelain will allow less of a color change. Although thin chamfer may produce improved color control, it is impractical because its thin porcelain margin makes it vulnerable in the dental laboratory or even in the dentist's chair. Hence a medium chamfer that allows color adjustments and porcelain margin of adequate thickness are preferred.

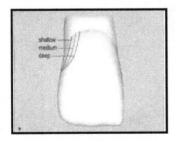 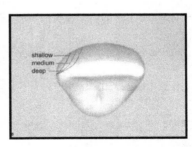

Fig- Ref- GUREL G. The science and art of porcelain laminate veneers. Quint pub.

Depth of extension

The palatinal extension of the gingivoproximal area is related to the required color change and the visibility of the area. Usually distinct color changes necessitate deeper preparations towards the palate. If the color does not need to be changed, the preparation margin can be kept shallow.[17]

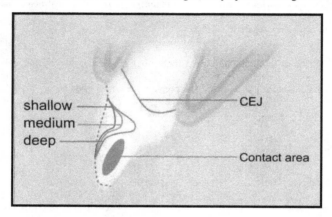

Fig- Ref- GUREL G. The science and art of porcelain laminate veneers. Quint pub.

Facial preparation

Based on the stratification method, 0.3 mm/0.5mm of enamel in the cervical one third is reduced blending this enamel reduction into the gingival chamfer.

Overreduction or underreduction is avoided by preparing until the depth cuts just disappear.

All the line angles are rounded off.

Incisal preparation

It ranges from 0.75 to 1.5mm depending on occlusal load.

It is necessary to terminate the incisal margin in such a manner as to protect against marginal peel.

This requires developing resistance form in the incisal preparation by either ending it at the linguoincisal line angle after reducing the incisal table more toward the lingual to provide added support to the restoration, or by ending it at the beveled facioincisal line angle to provide support from the incisal table of the tooth.

The reduction of the incisal table should not be done perpendicular to the long axis of the tooth but about 30°- 40° off perpendicular toward the lingual. This slight angulation toward the lingual provides resistance form against porcelain edge fracture and a sharp finish line for the ceramist to form a porcelain butt margin against.

If facial reduction leaves an incisal table greater than 1 mm in width & the length of incisors are not to be increased, then the sharpened facioincisal line angle can be given a 30° bevel, and the termination of that bevel on the incisal table serves as the incisal finish line. This alternative incisal preparation is a, reliable way of preserving existing incisal length.

If the incisors are to be lengthened up to 2mm and incisal table is less than 1mm in width, then the incisal table is reduced in a 30^0 to 40^0 plane toward the lingual until the incisal table width reaches 1mm or more. [23]

According to A. W. G. Walls et al. [6] decision about incisal edge reduction should be made during treatment planning. There are four basic preparation designs that have been described for the incisal edge

1. **Window** in which the veneer is taken close to but not up to the incisal edge. This has the advantage of retaining natural enamel over the incisal edge, but has the disadvantage that

the incisal edge enamel is weakened by the preparation. Also, the margins of the veneer would become vulnerable if there is incisal edge wear whilst the incisal lute can be difficult to hide.

2. **Feather**, in which the veneer is taken up to the height of the incisal edge of the tooth but the edge, is not reduced. This has the advantage that once again guidance on natural tooth is maintained but the veneer is liable to be fragile at the incisal edge and may be subject to peel/sheer forces during protrusive guidance.

3. **Bevel**, in which a bucco-palatal bevel is prepared across the full width of the preparation and there is some reduction of the incisal length of the tooth. This gives more control over the incisal aesthetics and a positive seat during try in and luting of the veneer. The margin is not in a position that will be subjected to direct shear forces except in protrusion. However, this style of preparation does involve more extensive reduction of tooth tissue.

4. **Incisal overlap**, in which the incisal edge is reduced and then the veneer preparation extended onto the palatal aspect of the preparation. This also helps to provide a positive seat for luting whilst involving more extensive tooth preparation. This style of preparation will also modify the path of insertion of the veneer which will have to be seated from the buccal/incisal direction rather than the buccal alone. Care needs to be taken to ensure that any proximal wrap around of the preparation towards the gingival margin does not produce an undercut to the desired path of insertion for the veneer. It may be necessary to rotate such veneers into place by locating the incisal edge first then rotating the cervical margin into position.

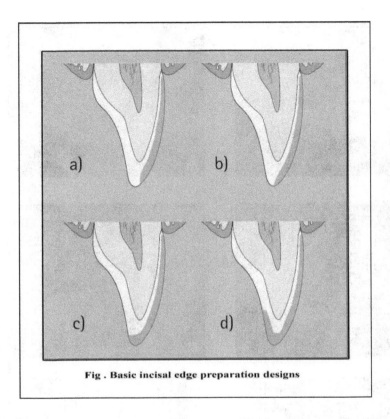

Fig . Basic incisal edge preparation designs

Fig- Ref- A. W. G. Walls, J. G. Steele & R. W. Wassell. Crowns and other extra-coronal restorations: Porcelain laminate veneers. British Dental Journal 2002; 193: 73–82

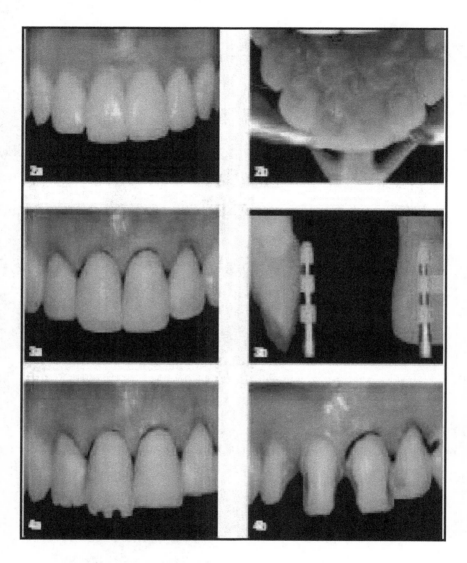

Fig- Ref- Philip newsome and siobhan owen. Ceramic veneers in general dental practice.
Part three: clinical procedures. International dentistry sa vol. 10, no. 3 (D-LD-Veneers-Pdf-
clinical)

Tooth preparation sequence: Mandibular teeth

Mandibular anterior teeth differ from maxillary anterior teeth in that they have thinner enamel plates, flatter gingival emergence profiles, require less esthetic emphasis in the cervical one third, and, most importantly, require disruption of centric occlusion and anterior guidance. Consequently, certain modifications are instituted for preparation of mandibular teeth to make provision for occlusal loading as well as contour and color correction.

Incisal clearance

To initiate tooth preparation for depth control, place two depth cuts in all mandibular anterior teeth. One depth cut of 0.3 mm is placed approximately at the junction of the middle and the cervical one third of the teeth from mesioproximal line angle to distoproximal line angle. The other depth cut of 0.5 mm is placed approximately 4 mm from the existing incisal table.

If the tooth makes contact in centric occlusion, take the tooth out of occlusion by 0.5 mm for mandibular incisors and 0.7 mm for canines, paralleling the plane of the existing incisal table insofar as possible.

The incisal table reduction will take the incisors out of occlusion by 0.5 mm and the canines by 0.7 mm.

A second preparation cut is then made, paralleling the facial surface, to the depth of the 0.5-mm depth cut. The intersection of these two preparation cuts will generally create an incisal clearance the facioincisal line angle of at least 0.75 mm for the incisors and at least 1.0mm for the canines.

For heavier occlusions, increasing the incisal clearance to 1.0 mm for incisors and 1.5 mm for canines may be advisable.

59

Gingivoproximal and facial preparation

The mandibular tooth gingival margin is not nearly as esthetically relevant as the maxillary tooth gingival margin. Therefore, for ease of impression taking and moisture control, as well as access for finishing, when bonding the veneers the gingival chamfer is routinely placed entirely in enamel, even if it creates a slightly supragingival margin.

The chamfer in mandibular incisors is not as pronounced as with maxillary incisors, being a maximum of 0.3 mm, because of the thinner enamel plate.

The proximal chamfer preparation is similar to that for maxillary incisors with the exception of the depth. It should be 0.4 mm as it extends from the papilla tip incisally to the embrasure. From the papilla tip to the tooth contact, the chamfer moves slightly lingually to hide the margin (dog leg effect) but remains just facial to the tooth contact to retain the contact in its entirety.

Cervical facial reduction for mandibular incisors is less severe than maxillary incisors, being in the 0.3 mm range. If a severe discoloration must be corrected by the veneer, approximately 0.1 to 0.2 mm must be added to the veneer to compensate for the insufficient tooth reduction depth, as suggested by the stratification method.

The facial reduction involves merely blending the middle one third of the facial surface with the cervical reduction and the incisal clearance reduction. This generally averages between 0.4 and 0.6 mm in depth.

All line angles should then be rounded.[23]

Finishing the Preparation

After all the steps that have been explained for tooth preparation have been finished, a thorough examination of the prepared teeth is necessary. The dentist must check to see if the incisal embrasures are opened, rounded and of varying depths.

Checking the Prepared Surfaces

It is preferable to check the margins under magnification. One final check should be made with the previously prepared silicone index from both the occlusal view and from the lateral view. This will ensure that the necessary reduction of the facial surface is done properly

Pre-sealing the Exposed Dentin

If any dentin is exposed during the preparation then it needs to be sealed before making an impression of the preparation. It's advisable to seal the dentin soon after preparation as there is superior bonding when bonding agent is applied to the freshly prepared dentin. It is done to prevent post-operative sensitivity and bacterial invasion of the exposed dentin.

Exposed dentin is etched for 15 seconds and rinsed. This should be followed by application of a hydrophilic primer which contains reactive monomer in an organic solvent, & can be more effectively used to prime the exposed dentin.

The frequent problem of bacterial leakage and dentin sensitivity experienced during the temporary phase can be avoided through the use of a bonding agent.

Etching

Etching time should not be more than 15 seconds. Longer applications will cause the collagen to collapse and negatively affect the bonding. If etching is done properly smear layer will be removed making bonding to dentin matrix possible.

Primer and Adhesive Application

Then the etched surface is washed thoroughly, but not dried. It should only be blot-dried with the help of a cotton pellet. While the dentin is reasonably wet, the primer should be applied and left there for a minimum of 30 seconds. It can then be gently warm-air dried from a distance. Now the adhesive can be applied over the primer & cured accordingly. [17]

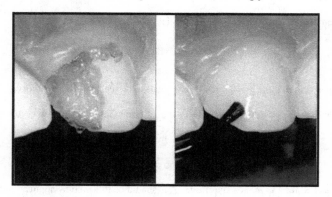

Fig- Ref- GUREL G. The science and art of porcelain laminate veneers. Quint pub.

Tooth preparation for spaced teeth

Because no space exists with spaced teeth, the proximal preparation is changed from a chamfer to a long bevel.

This bevel will terminate at the linguoproximal line angle and eliminate any proximal convexity that would create an undercut for a facial line of insertion. This involves carrying the gingival chamfer along the papilla tip until the linguoproximal line angle is nearly reached and then using the side of the diamond bur to flatten (bevel) the remaining proximal surface incisalward. The proximal surface is flattened by repeated passages of the diamond bur, until the long bevel reaches the linguoproximal line angle along the entire proximal surface. [23]

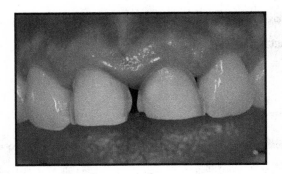

Fig- Ref- GUREL G. The science and art of porcelain laminate veneers. Quint pub.

Coping with pre-existing restorations

Some teeth that require veneers will have existing composite resin restorations in place. There are two ways to deal with this:

1. Bond to a prepared composite resin surface
2. Replace the restoration

Bond to a prepared composite resin surface-

Water sorption, exposed un-silanated surfaces of filler particles and limited opportunities for further polymerisation of the resin component of the set material all contribute to reduced bond strength.

63

Replace the restoration-

This can be done relatively easily, but should be done at the visit when the veneer is luted to the tooth so the new composite has the best chance of bonding to the porcelain veneer as well as the tooth tissue. This makes the procedure for bonding the veneer more complex. It can be difficult to avoid producing overhanging margins using this technique, so care is required to ensure that any such overhangs are identified and eliminated. [23]

Peculiar situations

Thin versus thick teeth

Thin teeth will be subjected to more bending stresses compared to thick teeth. Hence a thin flat tooth will require a substantial incisal clearance to generate a certain bulk of incisal porcelain. Conversely a thick curved incisor will require only minimum incisal reduction. [8]

Severe discoloration

Two modifications are to be made in the tooth preparation.

Location of the margin- it is the only indication for placing the margin slightly subgingival in position. Margin should not be placed more than 0.5mm subgingivally, since beyond this depth bonding becomes challenging.

More extensive preparation- to decrease the effect of darkening effect that the underlying tooth might have on the veneer, the depth of preparation should be increased. The labial surface should be reduced by 0.7-0.8mm in depth, with a cervical chamfer 0.4-0.5mm deep.

Lingual laminate veneers

Lingual addition of 'artificial enamel' by means of ceramic laminate veneers, although less common, may still be utilized.

Atypical teeth

Very pronounced microdontia sometimes occurs in lateral incisors. In these teeth, preparation will be very limited in depth and will encompass virtually the entire available surface. This is the only type of case requiring fine, knife edge margins.

Premolars

The labial cusp, whether maxillary or mandibular, should be reduced by at least 1mm, placing the occlusal margin away from the occlusal contact and grooves. The overlay extends to the occlusal three-quarters of the labial cusp, the margin being produced with a spherical bur and connected with the proximal margins by a rounded angle. [20]

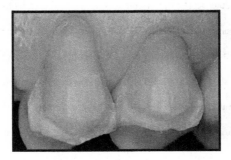

Fig- Ref- Touti B, Miara P & Nathanson D. Esthetic dentistry & ceramic restorations. Martin Dunitz. 1999.

SHADE SELECTION

To achieve a natural appearance details such as color, surface texture, luster, translucency and contour all play important roles in the creation of the ceramic restoration. A commercial color guide with limited selections cannot possibly cover the variations exhibited in natural teeth. Subsequently, any treatment must begin with first determining the color. The entire process of reconstruction and its success is directly related to the correct shade selection. Therefore, the technician must have all the related details to be able to make the precise and necessary adjustments. The enamel and body shades are selected in the same way. Color vision deficiency seriously hampers a proper shade selection. Therefore a dentist must be aware of any such condition, and if the condition is severe, they must use their assistant's or technician's trained eye to match the shades for them.

Importance of Light Source

Color is actually a phenomenon of light and a matter of visual perception that allows us to differentiate between similar objects. The perception of color depends on the object, the observer and the light source and our perception of a particular color may change when any one of these factors is altered. Perception of color is primarily influenced by light and so environmental light is very important. An interior shade room should be a part of any good dental office or laboratory and should be painted in neutral gray and be well light with color corrected fluorescent bulbs. The patient should not be wearing lipstick and their clothes must be covered with a gray bib. Only after these conditions have been met can the shade selection process begin. The ideal situation will exist if both the dental office and the lab have the same illumination sources as well as wall colors. This will minimize the metameric confusion.

Timing

The shade selection should be done even before the tooth preparation begins. This will avoid any value alteration during the preparation period (i.e. dehydration). In order to attempt to match the shade, the dentist must first be certain that the patient's teeth are perfectly clean and unstained. Consequently, it is very important to take the necessary photographs as quickly as possible, as even the simple procedure of using a cheek retractor for more than a minute is a cause for dehydration.

Stump Shade

Refers to all the shades of the prepared teeth after the reduction A common mistake during this procedure, that is made by most dentists, is to dry the prepared tooth surface before taking the stump shade. However, due to the phenomenon of dehydration, the color of the remaining tooth surface will appear lighter than when they are wet.

Low Value versus High Value

If a dentist cannot decide between two colors; it is beneficial to choose the lighter shade. It is always safer to go along with the lighter shade, as it is easier to darken PLV than to lighten it. (lower the value and increase the chroma)

Character of the Tooth

The three most influential factors are illuminant, observer and object. Careful recognition of these factors which include metamerism, gloss, translucency and fluorescence, will help to improve the result of the match. One of the keys to good matching is to recognize the tooth's original form, whether opaque, translucent, dull, or highly reflective. No matter if the porcelain restoration is brilliantly done or if the shade has been correctly chosen, if the surrounding teeth are dull, a high, glossy glaze will be incompatible.

Ocular Fatigue

If a color is viewed for an extended period of time, cone cells become fatigued and the signals to the brain thus decrease in accuracy of their perception of the object being observed. It can be difficult for the observer to distinguish between colors if ocular fatigue sets in. hence dentist should not stare either at shade tab or tooth for more than 5 seconds. Since blue fatigue accentuates yellow sensitivity, the dentist should glance at a blue object (wall, drape, card, etc.). The aged teeth need additional consideration, as their glossy surface tends to absorb any color close to them and thus distort the perception.[17]

Principles of Shade Selection

1. Remove bright colors from field of view

   - Makeup / lipstick

   - Tinted eye glasses

   - Bright gloves

   -Cover the clothing with the bib

2. Teeth to be matched must be clean

3. View patient at eye level

4. Evaluate shade under multiple light sources

5. Make shade comparisons at beginning of appointment

6. Shade comparisons should be made quickly to avoid eye fatigue(not >7sec)

7. Teeth to be hydrated [24]

IMPRESSION TAKING

After the tooth preparation is completely finished and the exposed dentin areas are sealed with the bonding agent, it is now time to make the final impression. Excellent impressions are a must. Without them the technician simply cannot produce aesthetic, well-fitting, veneers,

1) Soft tissue control - The periodontal condition of the teeth undergoing preparation should be carefully managed prior to the preparation and impression stages. Use of dental floss and interproximal brushes is essential to minimize bleeding, crevicular fluid seepage and to ensure accurate recording of the preparations and soft tissues and to obtain stable gingival height after the veneers have been bonded.

2) Retraction - Good impressions start with good retraction, but often the process is ignored or rushed and the impression compromised. Either single or double cord techniques can be used. A single cord is best used when preparing margins at, or above, tissue height, and where the gingivae are healthy and no bleeding occurs when the cord is packed. The double cord technique is best used when subgingival margins are required (most likely when deep discoloration is being masked). In double cord technique an extra thin cord such as#0 is placed into the sulcus following initial tooth preparation. This provides a slight tissue deflection allowing more access and importantly, it serves as a depth gauge to prevent cutting epithelial tissue. Once the preparation is completed a thicker, braided cord is placed to achieve adequate tissue displacement. After a minimum of five minutes the upper braided cord is removed, leaving the initial cord in place and the impression taken.

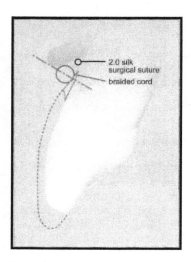

2.0 silk
surgical suture

braided cord

Fig- Ref- GUREL G. The science and art of porcelain laminate veneers. Quint pub.

3) Haemostatic agents - it is easier to respect tissue whilst preparing a tooth than to try and stop iatrogenically produced bleeding, there are occasions when gingival bleeding is an unexpected problem. Products containing ferric sulphate do not damage the tissues whereas commonly–used aluminium and zinc chloride products can be caustic to gingival tissues. all astringents negatively affect the bond strengths of adhesives to dentine hence use of cleaners such as a chlorhexidine, two percent glycolic acid or an EDTA-based cleaning gel may help return the bond strength to normal values.

Tray selection-

Selecting an appropriate tray for the desired technique and materials used is an extremely important, yet often overlooked, part of successful impression taking. Full arch, perforated metal, rigid plastic or custom trays are recommended to avoid inaccuracies that may arise when we take an occlusal registration, small double arch impression trays to capture the preparations, opposing dentition/occlusion and bite registration all at once are preferred. This method is often easier for the patient, since there is less material, a smaller tray and hopefully less risk of gagging. There is also the advantage of shorter chair time, since a bite registration and a separate opposing impression are not required.

4) <u>Impression materials</u> - A large majority of dentists currently use polyvinyl siloxane impression material. The material is easy to use, produces excellent results and exhibits essentially zero dimensional change during the setting reaction along with good tear strength and wettability. Most manufacturers supply heavy, medium and light body materials along with a very-heavy body material (putty) which is usually used to convert a stock tray into a custom tray for use with the wash technique.

Three impression techniques can be employed with the addition polymerizing silicones: the single mix (a medium body material is used in both the syringe and the tray); the double mix (light body in the syringe, medium or heavy body in the tray); and putty/wash (light body in the syringe and very heavy body in the tray). Putty/wash technique is very popular but prone to error as the putty invariably records critical areas of the preparation. [22]

Impression Making with Polyvinyl Siloxane

The impression tray should be coated with its special adhesive at least 15 minutes in advance. Before placing any material on to tooth the area should be kept clean of saliva, hemorrhage and sulcular fluids. The dentist starts applying the light bodied material with the syringe, which should have a relatively thin mixing tip nozzle, right over the gingival margins of the preparation. The aim should be, to try to place the material in between the gingival margin and the sulcus. At the same time the assistant loads the tray with the medium or heavy-bodied material. Once the application of the light-bodied impression material is finished, then the medium body loaded tray is seated (over the light body material) firmly in the mouth and it is held in place for seven minutes from the start of mixing. Once set impression must be removed as quickly and as straight as possible to prevent distortion. Addition silicones exhibit excellent recovery from deformation and they are very accurate and have high dimensional stability after setting. Then the impression is rinsed, blowed, dried, and then inspected. It should be placed in a disinfectant solution before pouring it. [17]

5) Complications from latex gloves - Some compounds used in the vulcanisation of latex surgical gloves may interfere with the polymerisation of polyvinyl siloxanes and thus contact should be avoided. For example, if mixing putty by hand, sulphur residue from the gloves contaminates the platinum catalyst and decreases the polymerisation reaction. Vinyl or nitrile gloves can be used to eliminate the problem. [22]

BITE REGISTRATION

In most of anterior PLV cases (unless the occlusion has to be improved or changed or if the patient is having some TMJ pain or discomfort) a simple "centric occlusion" registration will be sufficient. It is always preferable to have registration material that is as stiff as possible. It should be very soft when introduced into the mouth to prevent the patient from biting with force and forming different closing positions than normal. It is also wise to use a minimum amount of material in order to prevent the material flow into the undercut areas. [17]

PROVISIONALS/ RESIN TEMPORIZATION

Several factors need careful thought when considering provisional restorations including the need for them at all, technique and importantly the way the prepared surface is treated, especially if there has been any dentine exposure. As a rule, it is recommended that provisional restorations be placed for aesthetic and functional reasons. Aesthetically because teeth are often darker following tooth preparation and are reduced in size; functionally because interproximal and occlusal contacts need to be maintained and fragile margins need protection.[22]

The fabrication of the provisionals can be classified into two groups, as direct (intraorally) or indirect (extra oral) prefabricated provisionals.

Indirect technique-

- Prepared at the laboratory on a plaster, stone or epoxy model before or after the teeth are prepped.

- The technician approximately prepares the stone model and builds up the provisional mostly from acrylic.

- After preparing the teeth, the dentist tries to adjust the interior surface of the acrylic veneers for an easy fit over the teeth.

- Once the provisional can be easily placed, and then the inside of it is filled with a flowable composite and temporarily bonded.

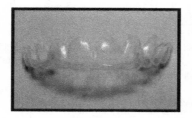
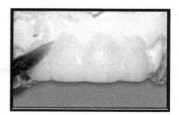

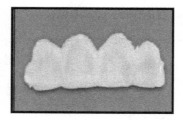

Direct technique-

There are various approaches for the different techniques.

Free Hand Carving

A very quick way to fabricate the provisional intraoral is by the freehand carving technique whether it is for a single veneer or two to four veneers. In this technique, the dentists have the maximum control to themselves.

- The tooth can be spot etched and the bonding agent applied and light cured.
- Then the necessary amount of hybrid composite, with the desired color that matches the adjacent teeth is rolled between the fingers.
- The material is then placed and shaped on the tooth, with the help of the index finger.
- If the surface texture or extension of the provisional to the interproximal is required, then special instruments can be adjunctively used and light cured.

- When preparing provisionals for single tooth, the adjacent teeth can be used as references in terms of length, tooth axis and color.
- If two to four teeth are being provisionalized, than the incisal length and position can be adjusted freely, paying the utmost attention to function and anterior guidance.
- The interdental contacts can be left separated in order to leave space for easy cleaning practices.

OR

- Coat the concerned teeth with water soluble separating media.
- Apply composite with spatula, remove the excess material and cure the composite.
- Now the provisional is taken out, shaped, adjusted and finished. [20]

Translucent Template or Silicone Impression

The second intraoral technique; is the fabrication of provisionals with the help of the transparent template which closely mimics the wax-up that the lab technician produced at the very early stages of treatment planning. [25]A thin vaccum formed acetate shell which is trimmed to remove the lingual surface and 1mm along the gingival margin of facial surface is used. [23]

- Once the teeth are prepared, they can be spot etched and then the adhesive is applied and light cured.
- The etched zone will provide an area to "spot bond" the veneers to place for the 1- or 2- week period until the veneers are ready to be placed.
- The bonding agent on the unetched enamel creates a temporary seal to minimize fluid contamination.

- The template is loaded with a flowable resin, with the color of choice and gently placed over the prepared teeth.

- After the composite is polymerized, if the provisional comes out, then the margins can be trimmed and polished extraorally and the provisional is then cemented over the teeth with noneugenol cement or with a flowable composite.

- If the provisional remains on the teeth, then the provisional is totally polymerized in the mouth and gingival flesh is cleaned with the help of the finishing carbide burs without violating the dentogingival complex.

- The final appearance is checked in terms of esthetics and function.[17]

Three application modes of the resin are-

a. One step, single mix (one single resin)

b. One step, double mix (transparent + dentin)

c. Two steps, double mix (dentin core/cut back + translucent)

One step, single mix

This is the traditional and shortest method. A single amount of core acrylic resin is mixed, loaded to the silicon index, and pressed over teeth.

One step, double mix

A small amount of translucent/ transparent mixture is first poured in the incisal edge of the silicon index. It is immediately completed with a second mixture of dentin like material and pressed over teeth.

Two steps, double mix

A uniform mixture of dentin is applied to the silicon index, which is pressed over the preparation until curing is complete. The incisal edge is then cut back to reproduce the natural morphology of dentin. Now the silicon index loaded with a translucent/ transparent mixture is pressed over the characterized dentin core. It results in highly sophisticated provisionals. [8]

In visualizing the many variables that will have an impact on the final appearance and esthetic value of the finished porcelain veneer, the ceramist will need to make use of all relevant information. Laboratory prescription forms, if used correctly, are an excellent communication vehicle between dentist and laboratory technician. They can provide all pertinent information and anecdotal comments. These accurate descriptions should supplement and accompany (1) a good impression, (2) bite registration, (3) cast of opposing arch, and (4) shade selection. Photographs are also an excellent aid to the technician. They can convey important information regarding the preexisting shade of the teeth, the lip line, the location and color of any discoloration or stain, and the relative position of the teeth, gingivae, and lips. [7]

Laboratory Communication

A solid collaboration between the dentist and laboratory is essential to achieve the desired esthetic result. The restorative team must work together (dentist-technician) to develop common goals, interests, and values.

Photography

Pictures help the technician to know the shape and texture of the teeth. Pictures make it easy for the laboratory technician to actually see the tooth contours, the translucencies within the incisal edge, hypoplastic spots, enamel staining and the actual intensity of the characterization.

Color Communication

The most sensitive and critical area of communication is that of color. It requires very close communication of concise information between the dentist and technician, in order to select the most accurate color. Ideally, the technician should be involved in the selection process along with the dentist and patient. When this personal contact is not possible, photographic images serve as the next best way to communicate information. Photo of a shade tab placed next to an image of the tooth, provides a lot of information about the translucency, texture and luster, along with the chroma, value, hue and the shape of the tooth. In order to correctly assess the color, the tab and the teeth should be on the same plane and placed edge to edge.

With color, communication of the translucency and texture are important parameters that play an important role in the value of the teeth. [17]

Laboratory prescription

A complete laboratory prescription consists of the following:

1. Shade(s) of prepared teeth: incisors, canines, premolars.

2. Shade gradation of veneers: cervical, body, incisal

3. Appropriate interface space in die spacer coats

4. Translucency/ opacity level of veneers

5. Veneer surface anatomy, texture, gloss

6. Veneer length, contacts, incisal shape [23]

When photographing the mamelons there will be too much reflected light if the camera is held perpendicular to the labial surface. To avoid this, the camera must be held high at a 30-degree angle downwards. To record the translucency the teeth should be photographed clenched and opened. The thickness of the enamel layer and any crack lines can be seen in the photographs taken at a 30-degree side angle.

Full-face Pictures

The photographs should not only be limited to 1:1 intraoral pictures, as full face pictures are very useful and should always be taken and utilized. This is the best way to communicate with the lab in terms of teeth and lip relationships and the relation of them to the whole face. Pictures should be taken before, during and after the preparation and the provisionals. [17]

LAB PROCEDURE

A key advantage of porcelain veneers is that they are fabricated indirectly in a laboratory. They utilize the ceramist's expertise in creating a realistic restoration yet still allow the dentist the opportunity to individualize and characterize the veneer through chairside shade techniques and cosmetic contouring.

Four diverse laboratory techniques for fabrication of porcelain veneers have gained wide acceptance:

1. The refractory investment technique

2. The platinum foil technique

3. Castable and pressed porcelain veneers

4. Milling systems- CAD/CAM and copy milling

The platinum foil and refractory die techniques are common choices because there is no need to purchase expensive laboratory equipment, and both methods are simple and can produce reasonably well fitting veneers. Both methods, if handled judiciously, will produce clinically acceptable, esthetic veneers.[9]

The Refractory Investment Technique

1. Fabrication of a Master Cast-

   A hard die stone should be chosen for pouring the master cast. Before this the impression should be treated with a liquid to reduce surface tension between the impression and the die stone and hence reduce occurrence of bubbles. The cast is allowed to bench set for 30 minutes. Once the stone is completely set, the cast is taken out of impression and allowed to dry.

2. Application of Die Spacer

A thin layer of die spacer is applied to the labial surfaces of the prepared teeth on the master cast. The die spacer should be kept clear of the margins

3. Fabrication of Refractory Model

A refractory investment material should be chosen with a coefficient of thermal expansion similar to that of the ceramic being used for the porcelain veneer. A preformed plastic disposable tray to fit on the master cast over the teeth to be veneered is selected. Only a labial-incisal impression is taken. The lingual flange on the impression tray and the tray material distal to the last tooth being veneered is cut. Master cast is surveyed for undercut areas & the undercuts are blocked out using oil based block out wax. Now the cast is coated with silicone-based lubricant. An elastic impression is made of the cast. Once the impression sets, both cast and impression is submerged in water. Now the impression is separated from cast and refractory material is poured in the impression and allowed to bench set. Once the refractory model is completely dry, the model from the impression is released while submerged in water. A second refractory model may be poured, following the same procedure used with the first refractory model.

4. Preparation of Refractory Model

The porcelain veneers may be built on either a solid refractory model or on individual refractory dies taken from two refractory models. Whether using a solid refractory model or separate refractory dies, undercut the die stem apical to the cervical margin, trim away the gingival area, and eliminate the interdental papillae. The finish line will then be defined distinctly. The solid refractory cast or individual dies are reduced below the gingival margin 13 to 19 mm to allow for easier handling. Minimizing the bulk of the refractory investment allows for easier handling. It also leaves less investment material to be de-gassed and facilitates a more uniform firing of the investment material and ceramic.

5. De-Gassing the Refractory Investment

To avoid contamination of the ceramic, ammonia gases inherent in the refractory material must be removed. Manufacturers' de-gassing procedures should be followed specifically for the chosen investment material.

6. Sealant Application

Done so that the refractory investment will not absorb moisture from the porcelain mix, a specific refractory sealant may be placed over all porcelain bearing surfaces and marginal areas. Any sealant or a slurried mix of the veneering porcelain can be applied to the porcelain-bearing surfaces. The sealant must be applied beyond the labial margins to achieve a good peripheral seal. Then fire the painted refractory model, or dies, according to the firing cycle of the porcelain being used. The porcelain is built up to full contour and the veneers are finished and contoured prior to stain application and glazing.

7. Removal of Veneers from Refractory Material

After the veneers are glazed and bench cooled, carefully trim the refractory investment material with an appropriate bur until only a minimal amount of refractory material remains around the veneers. Air abrade the refractory cast to remove the refractory material from the interface of the veneer. Carefully remove and clean the veneers in an ultrasonic detergent bath for three minutes.[7]

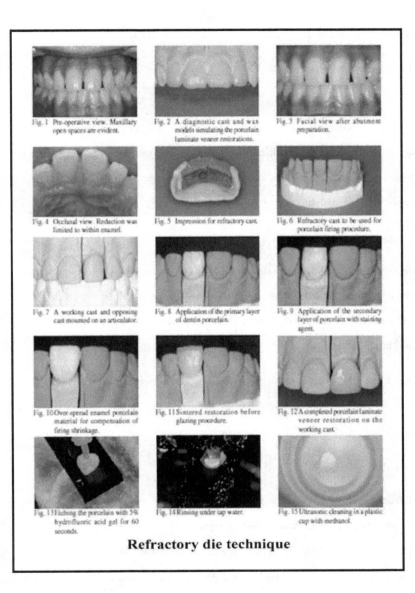

Fig. 1 Pre-operative view. Maxillary open spaces are evident.

Fig. 2 A diagnostic cast and wax models simulating the porcelain laminate veneer restorations.

Fig. 3 Facial view after abutment preparation.

Fig. 4 Occlusal view. Reduction was limited to within enamel.

Fig. 5 Impression for refractory cast.

Fig. 6 Refractory cast to be used for porcelain firing procedure.

Fig. 7 A working cast and opposing cast mounted on an articulator.

Fig. 8 Application of the primary layer of dentin porcelain.

Fig. 9 Application of the secondary layer of porcelain with staining agent.

Fig. 10 Over-spread enamel porcelain material for compensation of firing shrinkage.

Fig. 11 Sintered restoration before glazing procedure.

Fig. 12 A completed porcelain laminate veneer restoration on the working cast.

Fig. 13 Etching the porcelain with 5% hydrofluoric acid gel for 60 seconds.

Fig. 14 Rinsing under tap water.

Fig. 15 Ultrasonic cleaning in a plastic cup with methanol.

Refractory die technique

Fig- Ref- Garber D, Goldstein R & Feinman R. Porcelain laminate veneers. Quint pub.

The platinum Foil Technique

1. Choosing a Foil

Platinum foil commonly used for veneering is 0.001 to 0.00085 in. in thickness. the handling characteristics of different manufacturer's platinum foil may vary hence it is recommended that a foil designed specifically for fabrication of porcelain veneers be used. The platinum foil not only acts as a surface substrate for veneer buildup but also serves to radiate heat during firing, bringing the entire porcelain to a uniform maturity.

2. Model and Die Preparation

A good quality elastomeric impression is poured using a hard dental die stone to make a working model. Build up a base of at least 10 mm from the gingival margin and trim it when the model is set. A double pinning technique is used to pin all teeth to be veneered. Pour the base allow it to harden, and then trim it.

Section and cut individual dies from the master cast. Use a no. 8 round bur to undercut the die at the gingival and proximal margins. Cover all undercuts and enamel flaws with a block-out wax to facilitate easy removal of the foil

3. Foil Matrix

Cut the foil into the designated shape. Systematically wrap the foil over the incisal edge and into the undercuts of the gingival/proximal margins. An orangewood stick is used to adapt and burnish the foil into an intimately fitting form. The excess foil on the proximal surfaces beyond the margins must be trimmed away using a scalpel. An alternative process involves "swaging" the platinum foil. In this procedure, the foil is adapted to the die, lightly burnished, wrapped with a protective sheet of plastic, and positioned in a swaging apparatus. The die is dislodged from the swaging apparatus and the plastic wrap removed, leaving a foil very closely adapted to the die. To remove the foil matrix from the die, carefully lift the tab extension from the gingival surface toward the incisal surface in a hinge like fashion. Hold this foil matrix over a Bunsen burner flame until it glows bright orange, to decontaminate and anneal it. The decontaminated foil is then readapted to the die and secured with several peripherally placed drops of sticky wax. Mix and apply the preselected porcelain shades to the platinum foil. Fire the porcelain according to manufacturer's instructions. Complete the finishing and glazing.

4. Removal of Foil

By grasping the edge of the foil with the fine serrated-tip tweezers, gently pull the foil away from the veneer. Submerging the veneer in water will reduce surface tension for easier removal of foil. When the foil is peeled away from the interface of the finished veneer, the interface will have a smooth, glaze-like surface, not suitable for bonding. Therefore, it is advantageous to use a por-celain with optimum etching characteristics in order to develop an internal surface that will bond effectively to the tooth.7

Disadvantage with this platinum foil technique is that the margins of the dies easily get damaged during adaptation or swaging of the platinum foil and more overcontouring occurs with veneers fabricated on a platinum foil matrix, because the margins on the cast are being masked by the foil.[9]

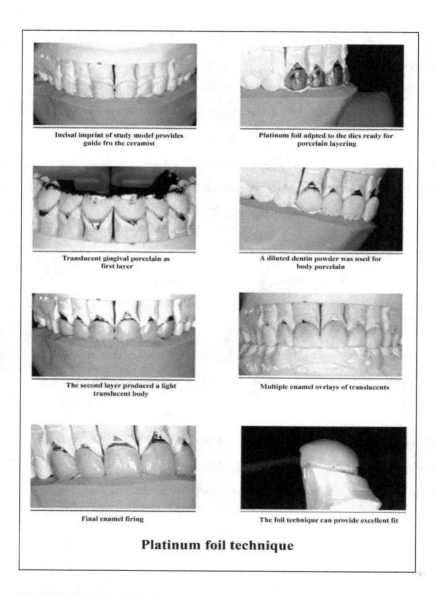

Incisal imprint of study model provides guide fro the ceramist

Platinum foil adpted to the dics ready for porcelain layering

Translucent gingival porcelain as first layer

A diluted dentin powder was used for body porcelain

The second layer produced a light translucent body

Multiple enamel ovrlays of translucents

Final enamel firing

The foil technique can provide excellent fit

Platinum foil technique

Fig- Ref-The Journal of Cosmetic Dentistry • Fall 2005, Volume 21 (3)

Cast ceramic laminate systems

There are two distinct systems of cast ceramic laminates:

1. Cast ceramic- Dicor
2. Castable apatite- CeraPearl

These two systems are very similar despite the fact that the procedures and materials are very different. In both systems, wax patterns are fabricated on a conventional working cast and die system. The wax is molded to reproduce the harmonious esthetic tooth form desired. These patterns are finished in their entirety, removed, sprued and invested in their respective type of crucibles, depending on the type of system being used. The crucibles are then correctly heated to the appropriate temperature and placed in their respective casting machines.

For Dicor system, the cast glass laminate is removed from the investment and placed in the ceramming oven; this process changes the external surface of the glass and crystalline structure.

For the CeraPearl system, the entire mold is transferred to the crystallization oven and heated at 870^0C for one hour. Crystallization takes place, producing a casting of hydroxyapatite crystals. The casting is then separated from the investment and cleaned, using the conventional sand blasting technique and alumina oxide powder.

The cast ceramic laminates can then be smoothed, polished, and tried into the patient's mouth.

Shading of Cera Pearl laminates is derived predominately from a resin system that transmits the color from below the hydroxiapatite veneer. Some alteration of the surface can be done with superficial stains.

The external surface of a Dicor laminate is shaded and characterized using the Dicor ceramic shading system and firing it in the conventional manner.[9]

Each system has its own particular armamentarium, and once the investment is set, the mold is placed in a burn-out furnace and gently heated to volatilize the wax pattern.

PRESSABLE CERAMICS

Pressed ceramics were developed to take advantage of the lost wax technique. Rather than casting the ceramic, a pressing process was developed which results in a molten glass pellet being forced into the mould created. This results in a very dense ceramic material that fits like gold and has high flexural and compressive strength. Pressed ceramics exhibit higher filler particle content, resulting in increased toughness (resistance to crack propagation). Because the outside surface of the porcelain cools before the inside, it develops a lower coefficient of thermal expansion, causing it to expand more. The resulting compressive forces cause a further strengthening of the porcelain. Higher leucite content also contributes to increased strength of today's pressed ceramics.

Here the ingots are heated and molded under pressure to produce the restorations. A full-contour crown is waxed, invested and placed in a specialized mold that has an alumina plunger. The ceramic ingot is placed under the plunger, the entire assembly is heated to 1150^0 C and the plunger presses the molten ceramic into the mold.[13]

CAD/CAM

Computer-aided design (CAD) and computer-aided manufacturing (CAM) technology systems use computers to collect information, design, and manufacture a wide range of products. Dental CAD/CAM systems have the potential to minimize inaccuracies in technique and reduce hazards of infectious cross-contamination associated with conventional multistage fabrication of indirect restorations.

CAD/CAM systems may be categorized as either in-office or laboratory systems.

In office ex- Cerec 3

Lab ex- Cerec inLab, Procera, Lava [16]

CEREC 3 has two-bur-system instead of the traditional cutting wheels or disks. The introduction of "step bur," has reduced diameter of the top one-third of the cylindrical bur to a small diameter tip which enables high precision form-grinding with reasonable bur life.[26]

The problem with the computer system veneers is the need to alter the color of originally monochromatic ceramic blocks with shade modifiers placed under the veneers or with surface stains fired over them. [9]

Debonding the Provisionals

In order to start the try-in, the provisional veneers have to first be debonded. A spoon excavator can help, by levering the provisionals from the proximal wall, which will pop off the veneer at the proximal margin. If the provisional resists dislodgment, then the facial surface can be vertically cut with a tapered fissure diamond bur. Before the try-in, one of the most frequently ignored stages is the careful examination of the tooth surface itself. The facial and proximal surfaces of the prepared teeth should be carefully examined for any residual resin cement or provisional resin leftovers. If residue is found, it should be carefully removed. It is of vital importance to clarify this, in order to enhance the perfect fit of the PLVs. It is always better to check it with the help of magnifying loops. [17]

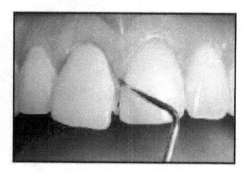

Now the PLVs can be tried in after the prepared tooth is first cleaned with fine pumice and water. The tooth must then be thoroughly rinsed to free the tooth of any traces of pumice. Any substances that may cause bleeding should not be used, as bleeding can be detrimental to bonding and, therefore, all use of powder cleaners or brushes should be avoided.

VENEER TRY-IN FOR INDIVIDUAL AND COLLECTIVE FIT

Initial veneer inspection

- Upon receiving the etched porcelain veneers from the laboratory, the dentist should thoroughly inspect each veneer to determine if any imperfections are present.
- The porcelain veneers are fragile before bonding and should be handled with care.
- Check each veneer for crack or craze lines.
- Then seat each veneer individually and check for marginal fit.
- After each veneer has been individually checked, seat the veneers sequentially on the master cast until all veneers are in place.
- Occasionally, an interproximal interference or an overextended margin will necessitate delicately modifying the veneers, with microfine diamond burs, silent stones, or rubber wheels.
- Do not force the veneers into position because they can fracture or crack.

Chairside try in sequence for individual and collective fit

If veneers are carefully inspected and the veneers are acceptable, the veneers are then ready to be placed on the patient.

We can now try-in the veneers on the patient for fit and select the resin cement to be used to achieve our intended veneer color. Basically, the try-in phase consists of three separate steps:

a. Dry try-in of each individual veneer for marginal fit

b. Wet try-in of all veneers collectively with a clear liquid medium, such as water-soluble glycerin, for proximal fit

c. Resin cement try-in of one or several veneers for color match to the appropriate color standard for the case.

Steps of try in-

1. Isolate the teeth with cotton rolls and/or lip retractors. Remove any resin provisional veneer by dislocating the resin near the unetched margins with a sharp instrument. Then spot grind carefully the bonded remnant of the temporary resin to thin it. Remove the remaining resin with disks, thus exposing the enamel without reducing it to any degree.

2. Clean the teeth with fine flour of pumice and remove interproximal surface contamination with floss.

3. Except where the margin is 0.5 mm supragingival or more, place braided retraction cord subgingival to prevent sulcular moisture or bleeding from contaminating the surface.

4. Try each veneer in dry to determine marginal accuracy. Adjust the veneer margin where indicated.

5. Fill the internal etched surface of the porcelain veneers with water-soluble glycerin to minimize dislodgement if a vertical position is assumed. Try-in the porcelain veneers in sequential fashion. If any porcelain veneer resists seating due to binding interproximally, remove the veneer. Use a microfine diamond bur or rubber wheels and carefully reduce the proximal surface. Reduction is delicately continued until the veneer seats properly. 30 fluted polishing burs, ultrafine disks are used.

Check the Color

After the veneers are comfortably seated, they should be checked with the shade evaluated under incandescent, fluorescent, and natural light. Before the actual cementation the dentist can allow the patients to moisten the ceramic and adjacent teeth with saliva and to observe themselves in a normal wall mirror for approval.

Try in for color

Place one central incisor veneer on the prepared tooth with either glycerin or a light clear try in gel. This veneer is used as a starting point for selection of the appropriate porcelain resin cement. If the stratification method of laboratory communication was used and a 0.3mm/0.5mm preparation was made for a two shade shift or less, the try in veneer color will frequently match the intended shade closely. If this occurs, then select the lightest translucent porcelain resin cement kit. Ideally, this resin cement would be virtually clear or colorless gel.

Color modification guidelines

Depending on the degree of color shift, i.e. one-shade shift or match color, two-shade shift, three-shade shift or more, certain general guidelines can be defined to select resin cement selection for any given case.

Matching color

To match existing tooth color or lighten the tooth one shade, a minimum opacity veneer is chosen to allow a significant portion of the background tooth color to show through. Hence the resin cement selection narrows to either a light, clear translucent cement, or a light, translucent resin cement

Modifying color

To modify the prepared tooth color by two shades, resin cement lighter than desired shade and with correct tint in color range of desired shade plus a small amount of opaque resin or opaque color modifier should be used. The ceramic used for veneer should have minimum to medium opacity- ½ to 1 shade lighter than desired shade.[23]

Masking the color

For a three-shade shift or more, to correct the color of profoundly stained teeth, a medium to maximum opacity veneer is requested that is at least one shade lighter than the selected shade for the case. Resin cement used should be opaque with tint to block discoloration and emphasize dominant color of desired shade.

Once the resin cement selection has been finalized the porcelain resin cement used on one or both of the central incisor veneers must be completely removed from the etched surfaces of the veneers. This can be accomplished with alcohol, acetone, or methyl chloride. Alcohol is preferred because of its lower cost and less toxicity. The veneers are initially cleared of gross resin cement on the etched surface by placing them, one at a time, in a dappen dish of alcohol and "scrubbing" the etched surface with a small brush. Then the veneers are transferred into another dappen dish of alcohol to remove any additional traces of resin cement remnants (no turbidity in the alcohol solution). Any residual resin cement that is tenacious can be removed by ultrasonic cleaning with alcohol, acetone, or methyl chloride for 2 to 3 minutes or by placing phosphoric acid etchant inside the veneer for 30 seconds and rinsing the veneer thoroughly with water.[23]

FINISHING AND POLISHING

Finishing and polishing the bonded veneers is extremely important. During luting margins of veneers should have been completely filled with the luting composite. This is crucial not only for the sake of preventing the marginal leakage, but also for the ability to polish the cement layer into a smooth margin. The finishing process of the veneer margins results in removal of the glaze from the porcelain. The removal of the glaze of the porcelain restoration during finishing, with microfine finishing diamonds, causes a slight increase in surface roughness at the cervical border. Finishing grit diamonds followed by a 30-fluted carbide bur and diamond polishing paste can be used to polish the margin area. Polishing under water spray produces a smoother surface. [17]

When polymerization is complete, excess composite be chipped off and a 30-bladed carbide finishing bur should be used to gently remove all remaining excess composite at the gingival margin. 15- micron grit polishing diamond is used to polish the interface of tooth/composite/porcelain. The final polishing of the veneer is done with a series of ceramic polishing points and diamond dust impregnated paste with non webbed rubber cups.

The edge of the rubber cup is brought to just beneath the free gingival margin to bring the junction between the veneer, composite, and tooth to a high luster, ensuring that this area does not become a repository for microbial plaque.

The lingual margin is finished with the LVS-8 to remove excess composite. Check the contacts with dental floss and make minor corrections with a yellow- banded Compo- Strip. Usually just a few back-and-forth motions will be effective. Incisal embrasures can be nicely polished with ultrathin discs.

The patient should return at weekly intervals to be monitored for tissue response. [27]

BONDING

Thin porcelain laminate veneers are bonded to the tooth surface using an adhesive and luting composite. Therefore, the strength and durability of the bond between the tooth, the veneer and the luting composite is what actually determines the success of the PLV treatment.

Chemically, tooth material, ceramic restorations, and composite luting resins are very different materials.

Treating the Interior PLV Surface

Acid Etching

Once the PLV fabrication is finished at the lab, the inside of the veneers should be sand blasted and acid etched with a 10% hydrofluoric acid and then sent to the clinic.

Acid etching causes selective silicate compounds dissolution from the surface. An additional property of the hydrofluoric compound is the surface activation of ceramic materials.

This acid etching can also be made by the practitioner, just before bonding.

The hydrofluoric acid on its own or together with the sand blasting will enhance the micro retention of the internal surface of the PLV.

The bond strength of the resin composite to the etched porcelain and the micro-morphology of each pattern are determined by the concentration of the etching liquid, the duration of etching, the fabrication method of the porcelain restoration and the type of porcelain that is used. [17]

The CeraPearl system uses a 2N hydrochloric acid that selectively erodes the glass matrix. The hydroxiapatite crystals are inert, so there is formation of series of pits and tags on the treated surface, which promotes mechanical adherence.

The Dicor laminate is etched with 10% aluminium diflouride or 10% ammonium. [9]

Checking the Etched Surface

Etching is done for 1 to 4 minutes depending on the concentration of the etchant liquid, fabrication of the porcelain restoration. After completion of etching the inside of PLV should be rinsed with a sufficient amount of water. The display of the inside of the PLV should be opaque over the entire surface. Any place that displays a less opaque appearance, than that area should be etched again.

Preparing the Surface

The internal surface of the PLV should be thoroughly rinsed and cleansed after the try-in. To remove any salts from the etching process, the etched area should be gently rubbed with a wet, cotton pellet and then cleaned with alcohol or acetone to remove any saliva or fingerprint contamination. Once the inside of the porcelain is contaminated with a try in gel, cleaning the surfaces with acetone will not suffice. This can only be cleaned with re-acid-etching. If the etched surface of the PLV is contaminated with saliva, the surface should be restored with a 15 second application of 37% phosphoric acid. The best result is achieved when the 10% hydrofluoric acid treatment with an etching time of 60 seconds, is done after the try-in. If this technique is used, there will be no need to further acid etch the surface with phosphoric acid.

However, if the surface has already been HFA etched at the laboratory prior to try-in, then the interior surface of the PLV should now be covered with 30% phosphoric acid, rinsed and dried.

Ultrasonic cleaning

After the etched surface is rinsed with copious amounts of water, a great number of acid crystals still stay deposited on the etched surface that may affect the bonding strength. Hence all residual acid and dissolved debris can be removed from the surface of etched porcelain with an ultrasonic cleaning in 95% alcohol for 4 minutes, or acetone or distilled water.

Silane Application

A fine layer of a silane coupling agent is painted over the internal surface of the laminate veneer after it comes out of the ultrasonic cleaner. Silanization of the etched porcelain with a bi functional agent provides chemically bonding to the silica. The silane group bonds to the hydrolyzed silicone dioxide copolymerising with the adhesive resin. The silane eliminates the polymerization contraction gap, which forms in etched, nonsilanated and unetched silanated restorations. Silane application is done for 1 minute followed by drying with an air syringe. This allows evaporation of the solvent.

Silane is available as 2 systems:

a. Single component system

b. 2- component system

Single component systems that contain silane in alcohol or acetone are the simplest ways to silanate. In 2 component system two solutions are mixed with an aqueous acid solution in order to hydrolyze the silane, which will polymerize to an unreactive polysiloxane and therefore it must be used within a few hours.

Adhesive Application

Once a dry surface is obtained after silanization, the adhesive of choice is applied inside the veneer with the help of a brush or a small cotton pellet. This could be done in a synchronized manner with the dental assistant while the dentist is applying the adhesive over the tooth surface.

The adhesive should be compatible with the composite that is being used as a luting agent. At this stage, the adhesive should not be light cured. As soon as the bonding is applied, the transparent composite luting agent is preferably placed inside the veneer.

Treating the Tooth Surface

The other part of preparation in this process to achieve maximum bonding is the tooth surface. Since the bonding will primarily depend on adhesion, great care must be taken to work under the cleanest conditions.

Rubber Dam

A partially sectioned rubber dam application is preferred while bonding the veneers. It acts as a physical barrier to oral fluids, moisture, tongue and cheek movements so that we can manipulate easily in the oral cavity.

Cleaning the Surface

The tooth has to be thoroughly cleansed before and after the try-in stage. The water-soluble try-in gels or the temporary cement over the prepared tooth surface should be totally removed.

Lazing the Tissue

If any tissue has grown over the prepared margin due to a small gap left on the provisional it should be taken care of at this stage using a diode laser.

Preparing the Exposed Dentin

Sensitivity can be reduced by eliminating or minimizing bacterial growth under restorations. The recommended agent for disinfecting the teeth was benzalkonium chloride (BAC) mixed with EDTA. Even 2% chlorhexidine gluconate can be used.

Cleaning

Until the preparation is visibly clean, it should be scrubbed. Antibacterial solutions then applied over the etched surface to act as a wetting agent and to decrease bacterial concentration, without having a negative effect to the bond strength.

Acid Etching Enamel

The tooth should be etched with 30%-40% of phosphoric acid. Gels are favored over liquids due to our ability to exercise more control over the application of a gel than a liquid. Different acids have been described for etching the enamel, 37% phosphoric acid as a standard procedure, 10%maleicacid and 1.6 % oxalic acid 2.6% aluminum nitrate, 10% citric acid.

Since the dentin is already sealed, etching will clean the bonded area.

Adhesive Application

After etching the teeth are thoroughly washed and dried. Dentin should only be blot dried with the help of a cotton pellet, in order to achieve "wet bonding". The primer is applied over the exposed dentin area, left in place for 30 seconds and then very gently dried until the carrier of the primer evaporates. Once the glossy appearance of the primer is achieved, then the adhesive can be applied on both the dentin and the enamel. At this stage, it is important that the resin should not be light cured until the veneer is seated over the tooth.

Bonding

After the tooth surface and the internal surface of the PLV are prepared, the PLV can be bonded to the tooth surface. A light-curing luting composite is preferred for cementation of porcelain veneers. The resin is applied with a brush to the inner part of the restoration. In case a highly filled composite luting agent that is slightly more viscous is being, it is better to use a spatula to place it inside the restoration.

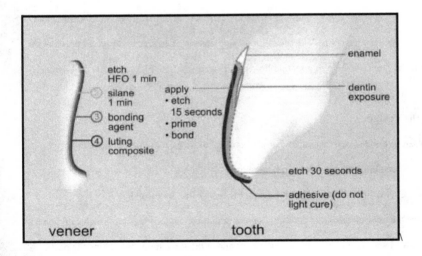

Fig- Ref- GUREL G. The science and art of porcelain laminate veneers. Quint pub.

Technique

When bonding the veneers one by one or as pairs, it is always better to place the luting resin inside the veneer to ease the control. A brush can be used to evenly distribute the composite inside the veneer.

The veneer should be positioned over the tooth very gently and slowly. Veneers need to be inserted starting from the incisal edge, and progressively pushing them towards the gingivoapical direction. It is one of the best ways of avoiding the formation of voids.

It is also very critical that the dentist must observe the luting resin flash coming out from all the margins, indicating that enough luting material is applied precluding any air residue of air inclusions in the bonding agent.

It is better to keep the veneer seated on the tooth with some sort of gentle pressure, either with the fingertips or with the help of instruments. The pressure should be spread evenly over the entire labial surface. It should be very carefully checked in terms of marginal fit, property seating and its relation with the adjacent PLV or intact tooth. Application of an apically directed pressure on the incisal edge with the help of a second finger will ensure that the PLV will have full contact with the tooth in the cervical area.

Seating the Veneers

Veneers can be bonded one by one, in pairs or bonding all at once. Diverting the operatory light from the preparations will eliminate inadvertent polymerization of the adhesive before veneer placement. Curing light is applied over the margins for only a few seconds.

This makes the excess composite partially polymerize into a jelly consistency which can then be easily removed without injuring the soft tissues, while at the same time minimizing the post-bonding finishing and polishing procedures. The inter dental contact areas and the gingivoproximal corners should be gently cleaned with the help of dental floss.

Light Curing

The resin is photo polymerized intensely after any excess is removed. To avoid the development of an oxygen-inhibited layer at the margins, an oxygen inhibition material, should be applied prior to the final polymerization. Then each tooth's veneer is light polymerized for 60 to 90 seconds on all surfaces. Once all the veneers are completely bonded, the rubber dam is removed and now the occlusion and protrusive contacts can be truly checked.

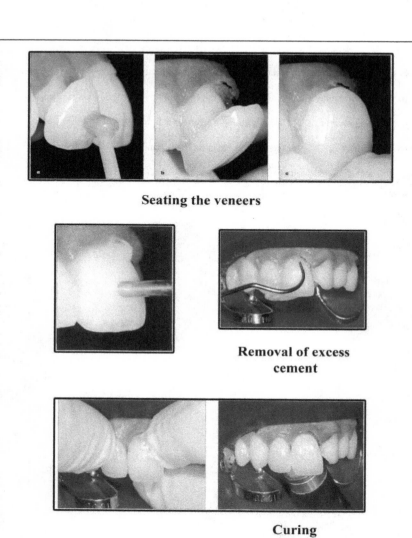

Seating the veneers

Removal of excess cement

Curing

Fig- Ref- BASIL MIZRAHI. PORCELAIN VENEERS: TECHNIQUES & PRECAUTIONS.

INTERNATIONAL DENTISTRY SA *VOL. 9, NO. 6. 6-16*

An instruction sheet should be given to the patient, explaining the do's and don'ts for the next 48 hours, as well as for the future.

Do's

• Use a soft toothbrush with rounded bristles, and floss as you do with natural teeth.

• Use a less abrasive toothpaste and one that is not highly fluoridated.

• Use a soft acrylic mouth guard when involved in any form of contact sport.

• Ensure routine cleaning.

Don'ts

• Avoid food or drinks that may contain coloring.

• Do not use alcohol and some medicated mouthwashes because they have the potential to affect the resin bonding material during the early phase (the first 48 hours).

• Avoid hard foods, chewing on ice, eating ribs and biting hard confectionaries and candy.

• Avoid extremes in temperature. [17]

CERAMICS COMPOSITION AND SURFACE TREATMENT PROTOCOLS [28]

Restorative Material	Composition*	Surface Treatment Protocols
Feldspar ceramics: Noritake EX3	SiO_2; K_2O, Al_2O_3, $6SiO_2$; Na_2O, Al_2O_3, $6SiO_2$ application	9.5% hydrofluoric acid for 2 to 2.5 min; 1 min washing; silane application
Leucite-reinforced ceramics: IPS Empress, Cergogold	SiO_2, Al_2O_3, K_2O, Na_2O, CeO_2, other oxides	9.5% hydrofluoric acid for 60 s; 1 min washing; silane application
Lithium di-silicate–reinforced ceramic: IPS Empress II	SiO_2 (57–80%), Li_2O (11–19%), Al_2O_3 (0–5%), La_2O_3 (0.1–6%), MgO (0–5%), P_2O_5 (0–11%), ZnO (0–8%), K_2O (0–13%)	9.5% hydrofluoridric acid for 20 s; 1 min washing; silane application

MERITS & DEMERITS

Merits

1. Natural and stable color. The smooth surface texture and natural color of porcelain are exceptional, and the crystalline structure of porcelain gives it optical refractive properties similar to those of translucent enamel. Porcelain can be internally stained and the ability to adjust the final color of the veneers during placement allows considerable flexibility in final shade adjustments. Texture can developed to simulate adjacent teeth, and this texture can be maintained indefinitely.

2. Inherent porcelain strength that permits reshaping teeth. Although porcelain veneers are themselves rather fragile, once bonded to enamel, the restoration develops high tensile strengths.

3. Extremely good biocompatibility with gingival tissues. The highly glazed porcelain surface is less of a depository area for plaque accumulation as compared to any other veneer system.

4. Long lasting. Once bonded, porcelain veneers develop high tensile and shear strengths and remain in place.

5. Exceptional resistance to wear and abrasion. They look good even after many years.

6. Resistance to stain. The highly glazed porcelain surface is very resistant to stain.

7. More resistant to deleterious effects of solvents, including alcohol, medications, and cosmetics than any composite resin veneer.

8. Lack of radio-opacity. On radiographs porcelain resembles natural tooth structure, allowing radiographic access to areas that would be shielded by radio-opaque restorations.

Demerits

1. Porcelain veneers can be easily repaired once bonded to the enamel, but the repairs are not long lasting due to staining which tends to occur at the margin of composite resin and porcelain.

2. The color cannot be easily modified once bonded in position.

3. Irreversibility of preparation versus little or no preparation for composite resin bonding.

4. Level of difficulty of fabrication and placement, time involved, and expense. The extremely fragile veneers are difficult for the dental laboratory to make and manipulate, and the process requires two appointments, and laboratory fees.

5. Technical difficulties in avoiding overcontours and obtaining closely fitted porcelain enamel margins. The margins can be especially brittle and difficult to finish.

6. Lower repairability compared to composite veneers.

7. Susceptibility to pitting by certain topical fluoride treatments. Stannous fluoride should not be used with porcelain restorations. [27]

8. If any cosmetic contouring or other adjustment be needed in Dicor laminates, because of the underlying white cerammed glass would be exposed. [9]

MAINTENANCE & REPAIRS

Bonded porcelain restorations have proved to be a very strong complex both in vivo and vitro. Medium to long term clinical investigations have demonstrated excellent maintenance of esthetics, high patient satisfaction, and absence of adverse effects on gingival health. As a result, the maintenance protocol barely differs from that applied to intact natural teeth.

Routine professional hygiene

There are no specific instructions regarding personal hygiene around BPRs. As far as brushing and flossing are concerned, the same care and techniques used for natural teeth can be applied to BPR- restored teeth. The clinician or the dental hygienist however must follow some specific guidelines during professional care.

Routine scaling

No mechanical intervention should be carried out in the absence of gingival inflammation and plaque.

Hand instruments should be used in a gentle tactile movement only when required. Careful movements should be made parallel to the gingival contour, and root to crown movements should be absolutely avoided, because they could easily chip the margin or ditch the interface.

The following devices should never be used.

- Sonic or ultrasonic scalers can significantly damage the ceramic (chipping, cracking)
- Air abrasive polishing systems harm the glaze, cause pitting and staining, and remove the luster.

Polishing

Heavy stains on accessible margins can be removed with silicon points or sonic brushes with dentifrices. Gingivally, placement of a deflection cord helps in this task. Dentifrice and a rubber cup can be used to polish the restored tooth.

Coarse polishing pastes must never be used because they can dull the surface of the porcelain.

Fluoridation

Topical fluorides, especially acidulated phosphate fluoride gels must not come in contact with the porcelain because they have an etching effect and can damage the ceramic surface.

Sodium fluoride gels are always preferred because of their inoffensive nature.

Complications and repairs

A preventive measure to reduce the risk of failure would be to provide the patient with a hard acrylic maxillary splint to be worn at night. Such an appliance is absolutely indicated for patients with acknowledged nocturnal clenching or grinding habits, with or without BPRs.

Postbonding cracks, chipping, fracture and microleakage are among the possible complications of BPRs. In most cases, repair can be made with simple means at minimum costs. The repairability of BPRs can also be attributed to recent developments of intraoral repair systems and tools. Among these, the intraoral sandblaster is the most essential device for ceramic repair.

Efficient Surface roughening can be safely obtained in vivo by sandblasting with intraoral sandblaster. A fine sand with 30um particles has been developed specifically for intraoral use. Because this sand has been modified with silica, it'll simultaneously allow roughening and incorporation of silica into the substrate, also called tribochemical coating. The silica enriched surface will then react with silane. Tribochemically treating the porcelain results in a significant increase in a significant increase of bonding characteristics.

Chipping

It's defined as a cohesive fracture that occurs within the body of the porcelain in areas of intense point loading. The pattern of this defect closely resembles enamel chipping found in aging intact teeth.

When esthetics and function are not compromised, the chipped surface can be selectively polished with fine-grain diamonds and silicon points and left as it is.

In severe cases, the lost fragment should be repaired with composite. Conditioning of the ceramic surface (sandblasting and Silanization) is required. The following procedure is recommended:

1. Isolate the dental segment under rubber dam to protect the patient's airway from sand inhalation.
2. Load sand into intraoral sandblaster.
3. Check efficiency on a metal strip.
4. Sandblast the chipped ceramic surface for about 15 seconds (neighboring teeth should be protected with a metal matrix).
5. Apply silane and allow solvent to evaporate (dry thoroughly with air and wait 5 minutes)
6. Apply adhesive resin, thin and cure.
7. Restore with light curing composite as for an intact natural tooth.

Fracture

If fractured BPR fragment can be recovered then it can be reattached.

Two scenarios can exist:

- The luting composite remained on the tooth, which suggests debonding at the porcelain composite interface. This could be the result of improper bonding (e.g., omission of adhesive resin to wet the etched porcelain), or improper use of silane coupling agents (e.g., insufficient drying)
- The luting composite remained on the ceramic work piece, which suggests debonding at the tooth- composite interface. This scenario seems to occur essentially when the underlying tooth substrate is dentin.

Postbonding cracks

These are more problematic because currently there are no procedures that can address this problem. if tolerated by patient, flaws must only be followed, and no specific intervention can be recommended at present. The patient must be informed that cracking does not constitute a risk for the remaining underlying tooth substance. Cracked BPRs should be replaced only in case of unesthetic flaws (deeply stained) upon the patient' request. [8]

FAILURES

Long term success of porcelain veneers can be attributed to great attention to detail in the following areas:

(1) Planning the case

(2) Conservative (enamel saving) preparation of teeth

(3) Proper selection of ceramics to use

(4) Proper selection of the materials and methods of cementation of these restorations

(5) Proper finishing and polishing of the restorations

(6) Proper planning for the continuing maintenance of these restorations

Marginal discoloration and loss of color stability

These problems occur rarely because

(1) All margins are in cleansable areas often easily finished and polished at the time of cementation

(2) The glazed porcelain surface, which is mostly impervious to extrinsic stain, also protects underlying light-cured (more color stable) resin cement

Causes-

a. Ill fitting veneers, which expose inappropriate amounts of resin cement at their margins

b. Well-fitting but poorly seated restorations caused by the use of highly viscous cements refinishing and repolishing can remove these dark lines.

If these lines are too deep, then a replacement restoration may be necessary. To remove excess cement series of trimming diamonds in a 30-mm, 15-mm, and 8-mm sequence of finishing diamonds can be used. This process is followed by finishing and polishing with strips and disks and then by porcelain diamond polishing paste applied with rubber cups.

Breakdown in bonds

If the veneer is not properly etched or if the veneer and tooth are in some way contaminated during the bonding process (i.e. water or oil in the air lines), it is possible to experience this problem or worse i.e. the complete delamination of the veneer. This occurrence is rare. Organization of steps at the time of bonding usually eliminates this problem. If a debonded but good-fitting restoration is recovered, the tooth may be cleaned of all old composite. The interior surface of the restoration can be delicately sandblasted and re-etched using hydrofluoric acid and then cleaned, silanated, and recemented.

Air bubble entrapment

Air bubbles can become entrapped near the margin of the restoration, which eventually becomes exposed. Food and other debris may be packed into the small space between the restoration and the tooth. The best treatment is first gaining proper access to this void with a pointed diamond and thoroughly removing any food and debris impaction. The porcelain can be etched with mild hydrofluoric acid and silanated, the tooth can be etched with 37% phosphoric acid, and new resin cement can be introduced with a thin syringe tip or compule.

Cohesive failure and repair

Another rare occurrence is the cohesive failure of either the tooth or the porcelain. The fracture of the underlying tooth is usually the result of poor judgment in selection of the tooth to be veneered. Vital anterior teeth with large existing restorations on the mesial and distal surfaces might be better served with full-coverage porcelain restorations bonded to the additional surface area of the crown preparation on dentin. Nonvital anterior teeth that have at least one surface with

117

large existing restoration and an average-to-large lingual access from root canal therapy should be considered for post core and full-coverage porcelain crowns.

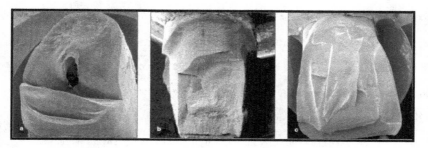

Cohesive fractures

A more common problem is the cohesive failure of the porcelain itself, which may occur during cementation as a result of a poor-fitting restoration, a resin that is too thick (viscous), or a resin that has gone through some initial setting. Cohesive failure also may occur after cementation as the result of poorly planned occlusion or traumatic injury. In the case of restorations that experience cohesive failure after cementation, repair may be attempted depending on the extent of the fracture. The following steps are suggested to follow for this type of repair.

A rubber dam should be applied. Resin block-out materials, can be used if a small area is involved but control of the field is necessary.

Sandblasting of the area to be etched is suggested, generally with 50-mm aluminum oxide particles. Roughening of the porcelain at the margin with a coarse diamond may suffice.

Hydrofluoric acid is applied to the roughened porcelain surface, which is followed by the placement of phosphoric acid on exposed dentin and/or enamel.

After following the manufacturer's directions on etch time, one should rinse and dry the surface

A suitable silane coupling agent is applied to the porcelain only

Silanes that come in two bottles that require mixing are generally best. Care should be used to ensure that the treated surface is dried properly.

After the silane has been added and dried, an appropriate unfilled resin or dentin bonding agent may be added to the porcelain/tooth interface and the excess is blown off the surface to be repaired.

This unfilled resin-covered surface is then light cured for at least 20 seconds.

Finally, a filled hybrid or micro-filled composite is placed, appropriately contoured, and cured as the repair material. It may be finished and polished to provide a smooth surface

Improper occlusion and its periodontal implications

Even a slight lengthening of the maxillary anterior teeth over the incisal edge can have severe consequences on the unrestored mandibular dentition because of the difference in hardness between porcelain and the natural enamel. If occlusion is not properly planned into the final restorations, it likely will result in longterm consequences. All cases should be articulated and checked carefully before insertion and final finishing and polishing should follow occlusal equilibration followed by protective night guard appliances. [5]

A clinical study was conducted by Bernouti Touti et al [20] on 170 patients for a period of ten years. The failures were categorized as mechanical failures (3.3%), biological failures (2.4%) and esthetic failures (11.8%).

The mechanical failures included split/ chip failure, cracks, fractures (try in/ bonding), and functional fractures (cervical, occlusal & debonding).

The biologic failures included sensitivity, microleakage, caries and necrosis.

The factors that lead to esthetic failures included visibility of margins (proximal, cervical), influence of underlying tooth, influence of bonding composite, influence of ceramic and build up technique.

RECENT ADVANCES

LUMINEERS

Advances in the technology of bonding porcelain to enamel created the possibility of porcelain veneers as an alternative to the use of full crowns for the treatment of many clinical conditions. Veneers were considered to be a more conservative treatment approach than full crowns because preparation of the teeth for veneers was thought to involve less tooth reduction than full crown preparations. Although this may be technically true, in actuality, the trend in conventional veneer procedures is to use very aggressive tooth reduction similar to that of three quarter crown preparations. "no prep technique," is characterized by little or no preparation of the teeth. In many cases, there is literally no preparation of the teeth, and in some cases, there is minor adjustment of the enamel at selected locations. The no prep technique was made possible by advances in custom-designed bonding systems and in porcelain technology that allow exceptionally thin veneers because of new exceptionally high strength porcelain. The veneers can be made with thicknesses in the range of 0.3 mm to 0.5 mm. In this thickness range, there is no need to cut down the facial surfaces of the teeth to accommodate the thickness of the veneers.[29] The success of each TPV case depends upon the results of the bio-esthetic prototype or mock-up. Viewing the mock-up allows you to give feedback for any modifications you might desire. Once the mock-up is approved, models and pictures are recorded and impressions sent to the ceramist. The mock-up is then carefully reproduced in truly thin, amazingly durable porcelain.

ADVANTAGES OF NO-PREPARATION CERAMIC VENEERS

No anesthesia required- Because only a small amount of enamel or no enamel is removed, these veneers can be placed without anesthesia,

Less patient fear- Patients fear the procedure significantly less when they learn that anesthesia delivery and tooth cutting are not mandatory for no preparation veneers.

Patients' appreciation of conservative tooth preparations.

Possibility of reversal- No preparation veneers are reversible, although it is seldom that any patient wants to return to the appearance of his or her preoperative smile. This characteristic makes redoing the veneers relatively easy some years in the future when they have to be replaced.

DISADVANTAGES OF NO-PREPARATION CERAMIC VENEERS

Overcontoured appearance- Because no-preparation veneers require minimal or no enamel removal, the teeth treated with these veneers are larger than they were in their natural state. The result is that the veneered teeth often have a bucktoothed appearance.

Possible need for more veneers- If the clinician is contemplating veneering only a few teeth with no-preparation veneers, producing an appearance that is harmonious with the patient's smile may require placing veneers on more teeth than those actually needing the veneers.

Opaque, monotone appearance- Often, thin veneers cannot cover discolored teeth without producing an opaque, monotone effect. Because of the minimal thickness of no-preparation veneers, it is difficult to cover objectionably dark teeth without the use of relatively opaque cements.

Limited translucence- The minimal thickness of no preparation veneers limits the clinician's ability to produce translucence in the veneers' incisal edges, as compared with thicker veneers requiring moderate-depth tooth preparations.

Margins not visible to the technician- If teeth are not prepared, the technician may have difficulty determining where to end the veneers, unlike when teeth are prepared for moderately thick veneers on which the margins are distinctly visible.

Possible overcontouring of margins- When margins of the tooth preparation are not visible to the technician, the ceramic must end on a nonprepared portion of the tooth. Because ceramic cannot easily be fired or pressed to a thickness much less than 0.3 mm, there is a tendency to overcontour the junction between the unprepared tooth structure and the ceramic.

Possible inadvertent alteration of occlusion- If the incisal or occlusal edges of the teeth are not prepared, there is a potential for extending the incisal or occlusal edges farther than the patient's occlusion can tolerate. Fracture of the overextended ceramic then becomes a potential postoperative problem.

INDICATIONS FOR NO-PREPARATION VENEERS

Small teeth. When teeth appear to be small for the patient's body size, and building them up to a fuller appearance appears to be logical, no preparation veneers are indicated if the occlusion will permit the anatomical change. An obvious example of this condition is "peg" lateral incisors, for which tooth preparation seldom is necessary before placement of ceramic veneers.

Anterior teeth with diastemas. If teeth are not too full in appearance and the patient has numerous diastemas, no-preparation veneers are a logical restorative choice.

Teeth in lingual version. Teeth sometimes are inclined lingually, producing an unpleasant, unnatural appearance. It is simple to correct this appearance by restoring the teeth with no-preparation veneers into a normal relationship.

Patient's desire for a change in teeth's appearance. Some patients desire to have their teeth made fuller in appearance and also to have the anterior teeth made longer.[30]

BIBLIOGRAPHY

1. I. Ahmad. Anterior dental esthetics: Facial perspective Br Dent J 2005;199 (1): 15-21

2. Sadowsky SJ. An overview of treatment considerations for esthetic restorations: A review of the literature. J Prosthet Dent. 2006;96:433–442.

3. Peumans M, Van Meerbeek B, Lambrechts P, et al. The five-year clinical performance of direct composite additions to correct tooth form and position. Part I: aesthetic qualities. Clinical Oral Investigations 1997;1:12–18.

4. M. Peumans, B. Van Meerbeek, P. Lambrechts, G. Vanherle. Porcelain veneers: a review of the literature. Journal of Dentistry 28 (2000) 163–177

5. John R. Calamia & Christine S. Calamia. Porcelain Laminate Veneers: Reasons for 25 Years of Success. Dent Clin N Am 51 (2007) 399–417

6. A. W. G. Walls, J. G. Steele & R. W. Wassell. Crowns and other extra-coronal restorations: Porcelain laminate veneers. British Dental Journal 2002; 193: 73–82

7. Garber D, Goldstein R & Feinman R. Porcelain laminate veneers. Quint pub. 1988

8. Magne P & Belser U. Bonded porcelain restorations in the anterior dentition: A biomimetic approach. Quint Pub: 2002.

9. Smales R & Chu F. Porcelain laminate veneers for dentists and technicians. Jaypee: 1999

10. Ching Chiat Lim. Case selection for porcelain veneers. Quint Int 1995; 26 (5): 311-15

11. Dino Javaheri, JADA 2007;138(3):331-7, Considerations for planning esthetic treatment with veneers involving no or minimal preparation

12. Choice of ceramic for use in treatments with porcelain laminates veneers. Med Oral Patol Oral Cir Bucal 2006;11: E297-302.

13. MA Rosenblum and A Schulman. A review of all-ceramic restorations.J Am Dent Assoc 1997;128;297-307

14. Ceramics update Journal of Dentistry, Vol. 25, No. 2, pp. 91-95, 1997

15. Michael C. DiTolla, Modern Ceramic Veneer Alternatives Director of Clinical Education and Research, Glidewell Laboratories Collaborative Techniques _ Winter 2003

16. Perng-Ru Liu. A Panorama of Dental CAD/CAM Restorative Systems. Compendium 2005; 26: 507-13

17. GUREL G. The science and art of porcelain laminate veneers. Quint pub. 2003

18. Ahmad. Anterior dental esthetics: Dentofacial perspective Br Dent J 2005;199 (2): 81-88.

19. I. Ahmad. Anterior dental esthetics: Dental perspective Br Dent J 2005;199 (3): 135-141.

20. Touti B, Miara P & Nathanson D. Esthetic dentistry & ceramic restorations. Martin Dunitz. 1999.

21. PASCAL MAGNE, URS C. BELSER. Novel Porcelain Laminate Preparation Approach Driven by a Diagnostic Mock-Up. J Esthet Restor Dent 16:7–18, 2004

22. Philip newsome and siobhan owen. Ceramic veneers in general dental practice. Part three: clinical procedures. International dentistry sa vol. 10, no. 3 (D-LD-Veneers-Pdf-clinical)

23. Rufenacht Claude. Fundamentals of esthetics. Quint pub:19900

24. Stephen chu fundamentals of color, shade matching and communication in esthetic dentistry. Quint pub: 2004

25. Seok-Hwan Cho & Won-Gun Chang. Effect of die spacer thickness on shear bond strength of porcelain laminate veneers. J Prosthet Dent 2006;95:201-8.

26. Werner H. Mörmann. The evolution of the CEREC system. J Am Dent Assoc 2006;137;7S-13S

27. Goldstein R. Esthetic in dentistry. 2nd Ed. Vol 1. Principles, communications and treatment methods. B. C. Decker. 1998

28. Carlos josé soares, Paulo vinícius soares, Janaína carla pereira, Rodrigo borges fonsec. A Surface Treatment Protocols in the Cementation Process of Ceramic and Laboratory-Processed Composite Restorations: A Literature Review. J Esthet Restor Dent 17:224–235, 2005

29. Schonfeld C. Lumineers by cerinate- The most significant advancement in 9000 years.

30. Gordon J. Christensen. Thick or thin veneers? JADA 2008;139: 1541-3

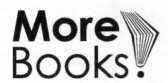
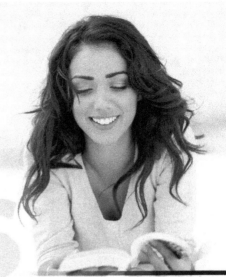
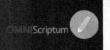

Printed in the USA
CPSIA information can be obtained
at www.ICGtesting.com
CBHW031258061124
17011CB00017B/41